GOVERNORS STATE UNIVERSITY
UNIVERSITY PARK
IL 60466

W9-BHM-738

Competency in Combining Pharmacotherapy and Psychotherapy

Integrated and Split Treatment

By

Michelle B. Riba, M.D., M.S.
Clinical Professor of Psychiatry, Department of Psychiatry, University of Michigan, Ann Arbor, Michigan

Richard Balon, M.D.
Professor of Psychiatry, Department of Psychiatry and Behavioral Neurosciences, Wayne State University, Detroit, Michigan

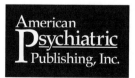

American Psychiatric Publishing, Inc.

Washington, DC
London, England

Note: The authors have worked to ensure that all information in this book is accurate at the time of publication and consistent with general psychiatric and medical standards, and that information concerning drug dosages, schedules, and routes of administration is accurate at the time of publication and consistent with standards set by the U.S. Food and Drug Administration and the general medical community. As medical research and practice continue to advance, however, therapeutic standards may change. Moreover, specific situations may require a specific therapeutic response not included in this book. For these reasons and because human and mechanical errors sometimes occur, we recommend that readers follow the advice of physicians directly involved in their care or the care of a member of their family.

Books published by American Psychiatric Publishing, Inc., represent the views and opinions of the individual authors and do not necessarily represent the policies and opinions of APPI or the American Psychiatric Association.

Copyright © 2005 American Psychiatric Publishing, Inc.
ALL RIGHTS RESERVED

Manufactured in the United States of America on acid-free paper
09 08 07 06 05   5 4 3 2 1
First Edition

Typeset in Adobe's Berling Roman and Frutiger.

American Psychiatric Publishing, Inc.
1000 Wilson Boulevard
Arlington, VA 22209-3901
www.appi.org

RC
483
.R465
2005

Library of Congress Cataloging-in-Publication Data
Riba, Michelle B.
Competency in combining pharmacotherapy and psychotherapy: integrated and split treatment / by Michelle B. Riba, Richard Balon. — 1st ed.
    p. ; cm.
Includes bibliographical references and index.
ISBN 1-58562-143-9 (alk. paper)
1. Mental illness—Chemotherapy. 2. Combined modality therapy. 3. Psychotherapy.
[DNLM: 1. Mental Disorders—therapy. 2. Clinical Competence. 3. Combined Modality Therapy—methods. 4. Drug Therapy—methods. 5. Psychotherapy—methods.   WM 140 R482c 2005]   I. Balon, Richard.   II. Title.
RC483.R465 2005
616.89'18—dc22
2004026974

British Library Cataloguing in Publication Data
A CIP record is available from the British Library.

GOVERNORS STATE UNIVERSITY LIBRARY

3 1611 00225 5526

Competency in Combining Pharmacotherapy and Psychotherapy

Integr~~~~~~~~~nd Split Treatment

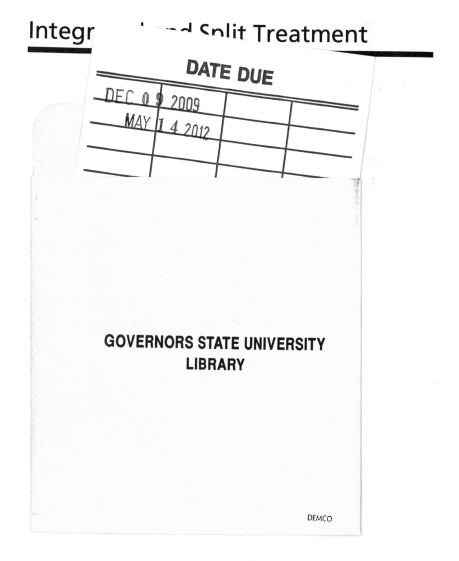

DATE DUE

DEC 0 9 2009		
MAY 1 4 2012		

GOVERNORS STATE UNIVERSITY LIBRARY

DEMCO

corecompetencies
in psychotherapy

Glen O. Gabbard, M.D., Series Editor

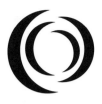

Contents

Preface vii

Introduction to the Core Competencies in
Psychotherapy Series ix

1 Introduction to Integrated and Split Treatment 1

Part I
Integrated Treatment

2 Selection of Medication and Psychotherapy in
Integrated Treatment 17

3 Evaluation and Opening in Integrated Treatment 31

4 Sequencing in Integrated Treatment 49

5 Termination in Integrated Treatment 61

Part II
Split Treatment

6 Selection of Medication, Psychotherapy, and
Clinicians in Split Treatment 75

7 Evaluation and Opening in Split Treatment. 83

8 Sequencing and Maintenance in Split Treatment 109

9 Termination in Split Treatment. 123

Part III
Evaluation, Monitoring, and Supervision

10 Evaluation, Monitoring, and Supervision of
Integrated and Split Treatment 139

Index 153

Preface

The practice of combining pharmacotherapy and psychotherapy for mental disorders has become the most frequently used approach to the treatment of these disorders. Most clinicians would agree that the combination of these two modalities is more efficacious and beneficial than each modality alone for a wide range of disorders.

Combining pharmacotherapy with psychotherapy may seem like a simple affair. However, it is a fairly complex process with many variations and permutations. Pharmacotherapy could be combined with brief psychotherapy, cognitive-behavioral therapy, psychodynamic psychotherapy, supportive therapy, interpersonal therapy, and many others. The combination of pharmacotherapy and psychotherapy could be delivered by one person (integrated treatment) or by two or more persons (collaborative or split treatment). The combination of these two modalities could begin with either pharmacotherapy or psychotherapy, with the second modality starting later. All these issues need to be factored in when considering combining pharmacotherapy and psychotherapy. The Residency Review Committee for Psychiatry appropriately decided that psychiatry residents must be able to demonstrate competency in combining psychotherapy with pharmacotherapy.

This book is intended to be a basic text for residents and teaching faculty in addressing competency in combining psychotherapy and pharma-

We thank Linda Gacioch for her invaluable help with the preparation of this book.

cotherapy. It is meant to be simple, straightforward, clinically oriented, and easy to read.

We feel that each psychiatry resident should become competent in and master both major approaches to combining psychotherapy and pharmacotherapy—integrated and split treatment—because these are common clinical practices.

Therefore, this book is divided into two major parts, the first dealing with integrated treatment and the second focused on split treatment. Some parts of the text in these two sections could, in fact, be similar if not identical, because they deal with similar problems. The resident, however, should read both sections of the book separately to familiarize and educate himself or herself with each particular treatment modality (i.e., integrated and split treatment). Each section is a separate unit standing on its own, and therefore should be read as such.

We hope that this book will help all residents in psychiatry to master and become competent in combining pharmacotherapy and psychotherapy. Ultimately, their mastery of and competency in this crucial therapeutic area will help to improve the lives of patients.

Richard Balon, M.D.
Michelle B. Riba, M.D., M.S.

Introduction to the Core Competencies in Psychotherapy Series

With the extraordinary progress in the neurosciences and psychopharmacology in recent years, some psychiatric training programs have de-emphasized psychotherapy education. Many residents and educators have decried the loss of the "mind" in the increasing emphasis on the biological basis of mental illness and the shift toward somatic treatments as the central therapeutic strategy in psychiatry. This shift in emphasis has been compounded by the common practice in our managed care era of "split treatment," meaning that psychiatrists are often relegated to seeing the patient for a brief medication management session, while the psychotherapy is conducted by a mental health professional from another discipline. This shift in emphasis has created considerable concern among both psychiatric educators and the consumers of psychiatric education—the residents themselves.

The importance of psychotherapy in the training of psychiatrists has recently been reaffirmed, however, as a result of the widespread movement toward the establishment of core competencies throughout all medical specialties. In 1999 both the Accreditation Council for Graduate Medical Education (ACGME) and the American Board of Medical Specialties (ABMS) recognized that a set of organizing principles was necessary to measure competence in medical education. These six principles—patient care, medical knowledge, interpersonal and communication skills, practice-based learning and improvement, professionalism, and systems-based practice—are now collectively referred to as the *core competencies* in medical education.

This movement within medical education was a direct consequence of a broader movement launched by the U.S. Department of Education approximately 20 years ago. All educational projects, including those involving accreditation, had to develop outcome measures. Those entrusted with the training of physicians were no exception.

Like all medical specialties, psychiatry has risen to the occasion by making attempts to translate the notion of core competencies into meaningful psychiatric terms. The inherent ambiguity of a term like "competence" has sparked much discussion among psychiatric educators. Does the term mean that practitioners are sufficiently skilled that one would refer a family member to them for treatment without hesitation? Or does the term imply rudimentary knowledge and practice that would ensure a reasonable degree of safety? These questions are not yet fully resolved. The basic understanding of what is meant by core competencies will be evolving over the next few years as various groups within medicine and psychiatry strive to articulate reasonable standards for educators.

As of July 2002, the Psychiatry Residency Review Committee (RRC) mandated that all psychiatric residency training programs must begin implementing the six core competencies in clinical and didactic curricula. Those programs that fail to do so may receive citations when they undergo accreditation surveys. This mandate also requires training directors to develop more sophisticated means of evaluating the progress and learning of residents in their programs.

As part of the process of adapting the core competencies to psychiatry, the Psychiatry RRC felt that reasonable competence in five different forms of psychotherapy—long-term psychodynamic psychotherapy, supportive psychotherapy, cognitive behavioral psychotherapy, brief psychotherapy, and psychotherapy combined with psychopharmacology—should be an outcome of a good psychiatric education for all psychiatric residents.

Many training programs have had to scramble to find faculty who are well trained in these modalities and teaching materials to facilitate the learning process. American Psychiatric Publishing, Inc., felt that the publication of basic texts in each of the five mandated areas would be of great value to training programs. So in 2002 Dr. Robert Hales, editor-in-chief at American Psychiatric Publishing, appointed me to be the series editor of a new line of five books. This series is titled Core Competencies in Psychotherapy and features five brief texts by leading experts in each of the psychotherapies. Each volume covers the key principles of practice in the treatment and also suggests ways to evaluate whether residents have been trained to a level of competence in each of the therapies. (For more information about the books in this series and their availability, please visit www.appi.org.)

True expertise in psychotherapy requires many years of experience with skilled supervision and consultation. However, the basic tools can be learned during residency training so that freshly minted psychiatrists are prepared to deliver necessary treatments to the broad range of patients they encounter.

These books will be valuable adjuncts to the traditional methods of psychotherapy education: supervision, classroom teaching, and clinical experience with a variety of patients. We feel confident that mastery of the material in these five volumes will constitute a major step in the acquisition of competency in psychotherapy and, ultimately, the compassionate care of patients who come to us for help.

Glen O. Gabbard, M.D., Series Editor
Brown Foundation Chair of Psychoanalysis
Professor of Psychiatry
Department of Psychiatry and Behavioral Sciences
Director, Baylor Psychiatry Clinic
Baylor College of Medicine
Houston, Texas

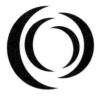

Introduction to Integrated and Split Treatment

In the past 10 years, psychiatric practice for most mental disorders in the United States has been increasingly characterized by psychopharmacological treatment (Olfson et al. 1999, 2002; West et al. 2003). Although for many psychiatrists in the United States the provision of psychotherapy may not be profitable, evidence-based practice guidelines (Lohr 1990) recommend that psychotherapy be provided for patients with many major mental disorders treated by psychiatrists, such as schizophrenia, bipolar disorder, and major depression (American Psychiatric Association 1994, 1997, 2000). Furthermore, evidence shows that patients who receive both psychopharmacological treatment and psychotherapy may have better treatment outcomes than patients who receive only psychopharmacological treatment (West et al. 2003) for major depression (Keller et al. 2000), dysthymia (Dunner et al. 1996), anxiety (Barlow et al. 2000; Mavissakalian 1993), bipolar disorder (Clarkin et al. 1998), and nicotine dependence (U.S. Department of Health and Human Services 2000).

For the major mental disorders for which evidence-based psychosocial treatments (both psychotherapy and pharmacotherapy) are available, it is important that psychiatry residents be able to provide the appropriate type of treatment (or combination of treatments) to the patient with the appropriate diagnosis. Furthermore, because this is such an important part of psychiatric practice, it is important that psychiatry residency training programs be able to document residents' competence (Epstein and Hundert 2002) specifically regarding the mastery of skills for psychotherapy and psychopharmacology, either by having residents conduct both treatments themselves or by having them collaborate with other mental health professionals as well as receive supervision on their cases.

One of the major challenges, however, has been combining psychotherapy and psychopharmacology: determining which professionals should provide the specific kind of treatment; timing and staging of the combination of treatments (i.e., which modality to start first or starting both at the same time). We begin with probably the most complex issue: how the patient presents for treatment, and how the patient's presentation affects the provision of psychotherapy, psychopharmacology, neither, or both.

Psychiatric Triage: The System Has Become Confusing

Psychiatric triage has indeed become very confusing and complex for both patients and clinicians. No longer are most patients able to call a psychiatrist or therapist directly and make an appointment for an evaluation. More often than not, patients are required call an intake worker via their managed care or insurance provider, give historical and symptom information over the telephone, and then be told where to go for an evaluation. If the symptoms are not acute, the patient may first be seen by a nonphysician (therapist), who will decide whether or not the patient should be seen by a physician for medication or other medical input. The decision regarding medication might be made at the initial evaluation or sometime later. If the therapist continues to see the patient for psychotherapy and the physician provides psychotropic medication, the physician is considered the *prescribing psychiatrist*, and the treatment is called **split treatment.** Of course, the prescribing physician can be a primary care physician or other physician. Some have used the term *collaborative treatment* (Riba and Balon 1999), but we prefer to use the term *split treatment*, because although the care should be collaborative—as all care should be—*split treatment* better captures the fragmentation that does occur in this type of care system.

If the patient sees a psychiatrist for the initial evaluation and remains with the psychiatrist for both psychotherapy and psychotropic medication, this is called **integrated treatment.** Similarly, if the patient is initially triaged to a therapist and is then referred to a psychiatrist who takes over both the psychotherapy and medication, this would also be integrated care.

Also, in many states, nurse practitioners and physician assistants are able to prescribe medications under the supervision of a physician. Therefore, a psychiatrist may be the supervising psychiatrist, not the treating psychiatrist, for patients who are under the care of nurse practitioners and physician assistants. In addition, at the time of this writing, New Mexico and Louisiana have given prescribing privileges to psychologists, with the details of the prescribing to be worked out by various boards of professionals. The role of psychiatrists in providing supervision or oversight in these states is still unclear.

What is so confusing about these forms of split versus integrated care? Following are some of the issues:

- There are no recognized guidelines for determining the best types of care based on symptoms.
- There are no recognized guidelines for determining the best types of care based on diagnosis.
- There are no recognized guidelines for determining the best types of care based on factors such as age, gender, and comorbid psychiatric or medical disorders.
- Triage is mostly based on insurance or ability to pay.
- Many managed behavioral-care intermediaries are judged according to the number of days that elapse before patients are seen after their initial call for help. This system encourages patients to be seen by the first available clinician rather than necessarily by the best clinician for that particular patient.
- Most insurance plans impose limits on the total number of psychotherapy or psychopharmacology encounters in a certain time period, which may produce tensions and negotiations between the patient and treating specialist or between the psychiatrist and mental health worker (e.g., would it be better to use these benefits for psychotherapy?). Some insurance companies complicate the process even more by not allowing patients to have a psychotherapy session and a medication review on the same day.
- Patients do not necessarily get what they want. They may want to see a psychiatrist, for example, but based on the symptoms for which they are presenting they will not see a psychiatrist, at least initially.
- Much of the triage is done over the telephone by workers from a wide variety of backgrounds, not necessarily licensed mental health practitioners.
- Countertransferential or other issues (such as financial factors or competition between clinicians) might arise in the initial triage or evaluation situation that are then imposed on the patient.

- Little research on outcomes has been conducted based on the above-mentioned nonstandardized procedures.
- There is little collaboration between the professions (psychiatry, psychology, social work, primary care) on the best ways to triage and manage the issues of split versus integrated treatments.
- The issues of split versus integrated treatment have been better studied in the outpatient setting. The role of the psychiatry resident on the psychiatry inpatient unit with regard to these issues has been less well studied during the past 10 years. The focus of psychiatry inpatient services has moved more to acute care and to rapid evaluation, assessment, and discharge, and far less psychotherapy is provided by residents than in previous decades.
- The role of the primary care physician as gatekeeper for diagnosing and triaging patients for psychotherapy and pharmacotherapy continues to be a major and important area of study. It continues to be difficult for primary care physicians to sort out psychiatric symptoms in the short amount of face-to-face time they have with patients. The physical symptoms with which patients often present (back pain, headache, fatigue, etc.) are difficult to distinguish from depressive and anxiety symptoms. Furthermore, it is often a challenge for primary care physicians to arrange for patients to be seen by qualified mental health professionals in a timely fashion.
- Psychiatry is undergoing increased specialization (geriatrics, child and adolescent, substance use, forensics, psychosomatic medicine), which contributes to the complexity of deciding between integrated and split treatment. Furthermore, guidelines for making the choice are still lacking.

The issues listed above are complex and not easily answerable. We suggest the following as a competency:

> **Competency:** Psychiatry residents shall demonstrate an appreciation for the triage system that is in place at their institution for both inpatient and outpatient psychotherapy and psychopharmacological treatments.

As illustrated in this chapter, even the initial triage system that begins the entry or route for the patient is complex. For convenience or logistics, the patient might want to see just one clinician for both medication and psychotherapy, but because of the nature of the system will end up seeing two clinicians. Because this arrangement may or may not be less expensive than seeing one clinician (Dewan 1999; Goldman et al. 1998), health care costs might not be the primary driving agent for this type of care.

The patient might see a social worker or a psychologist for the initial evaluation. The category of professional initially seen by the patient does not often follow a consistent pattern; the key factor might be whoever has availability or whichever type of clinician the behavioral system has designated for the role. Regarding psychotropic medication, the therapist might refer the patient to a psychiatrist or a primary care physician. Again, there are generally no standards of care that dictate the kind of physician who should or would be the prescribing physician.

The therapist and the physician might have a history of working with one another or not. The system of care might be closed, meaning that the clinicians in the system know each other, work with one another, etc. Examples of closed systems would be a university outpatient psychiatry clinic or a community mental health clinic. Alternatively, the system might be open in that the clinicians do not regularly collaborate with one another. Factors might include geography: if a patient is in an area where there is an abundance of therapists but very few psychiatrists or primary care clinicians, the patient might have to travel a long distance to receive care from a physician. In such a case, there might be less of a chance that the therapist and physician have worked together. Similarly, in an area with a large population of therapists and physicians, there may be less of a chance that the clinicians have worked together.

Added to these factors are many others that make the triage—and therefore the decision about split versus integrated care—very confusing and complex. Is the patient a child, an adolescent, or an older adult? Does the patient have a comorbid medical condition that would affect whether it would be best for the patient to receive both psychotherapy and medication in an integrated care model? Does the patient have a substance use problem? Are there psychosocial factors, family issues, a history of adherence to treatment, or belief systems regarding psychotherapy or medication that might have an impact on whether split treatment or integrated treatment would be best for the patient? What personal or other factors would be important for the clinician to understand in the triage process?

Competency: The psychiatry resident should be able to demonstrate the ability to take a history regarding factors that would have an impact on the decision to provide the patient with split versus integrated treatment.

Thinking About Integrated Treatment Versus Split Treatment

Why are the issues outlined above under "Psychiatric Triage: The System Has Become Confusing" so important and at the same time so vexing? The pathway for a patient to obtain evaluation by a clinician is no longer straightforward and is very dependent on a host of factors, many of which are not clinically important but are more dependent on fiscal, geographic, and insurance considerations. It is therefore incumbent on the psychiatry resident to take heed of these factors in trying to understand and then assess what is best for the patient regarding split versus integrated treatment.

Given that there are currently no standards or guidelines for determining these issues for patients based on age, diagnostic categories, comorbidities, etc., how should the resident begin to differentiate and think about choosing between integrated and split treatment for a specific patient? This is especially germane, because it is unlikely that the resident is conducting the initial telephone evaluation or triage and may be picking up the patient's case at some point after psychotherapy has already been started by another therapist.

Because this confusing system of triage and evaluation is becoming the norm in today's current psychiatric practice—in managed care settings, community mental health settings, and even in university ambulatory care settings—it is very important that the psychiatry resident be armed with the tools to understand the issues. Furthermore, besides understanding, it is necessary to provide ways to determine competency regarding both split treatment and integrated treatment on the part of the general psychiatry resident by the time of graduation.

The *Residency Review Committee* of the Accreditation Council for Graduate Medical Education (American Medical Association 2004) has published requirements regarding competencies in five areas of psychotherapy. In all these areas of psychotherapy, the general resident must demonstrate competency by the time of graduation. Each residency program must develop a method of testing and evaluating residents on the demonstration of ability and mastery of these forms of psychotherapy. One of these areas is psychotherapy combined with psychopharmacology. The Residency Review Committee is nondirective as to whether psychotherapy and psychopharmacology are provided in the integrated treatment model (psychiatrist or other physician providing both the psychotherapy and medication) or in the split treatment model (a nonphysician therapist and psychiatrist or other physician).

In this book, therefore, we provide guidelines to assess the competency of residents to provide both split treatment and integrated treatment. We believe it is important that psychiatry residents be able to understand the principles, issues, factors, and dynamics that underlie the confusing and complex panoply of ways that patients enter the psychiatric system for evaluation and that affect whether patients remain in split treatment or integrated treatment.

As an example, a patient may change jobs while undergoing split treatment with a therapist and a psychiatrist. The new employer's insurance provider could dictate that the patient change providers and might need to be seen by just one clinician. The patient might then decide to be seen by just the psychiatrist for integrated treatment. The psychiatrist must be able to adjust the care accordingly. Similarly, a patient might be in split treatment and not be doing well clinically. The psychiatrist must be able to determine the causes for this situation and determine if the patient would be best managed with integrated treatment. The psychiatrist, therefore, must be able to manage patients, understand factors, and easily move between integrated and split treatment. The competencies for both integrated and split treatment by a psychiatry resident must be taught throughout residency and evaluated by the time of graduation.

We also mainly focus on competencies in adult psychiatry in the outpatient setting. We recognize that inpatient units also provide split treatment. Certain patient populations (children, older patients) require split treatment in a different and unique format because parents and other medical professionals and caregivers are involved and because different types of consent and cognitive issues are germane, among other reasons. There are also certain diagnostic categories (e.g., substance abuse, psychosomatic medicine, forensics) that lend themselves to different types of split treatment, which call for unique competencies. The scope of this book is therefore limited to adult outpatient psychiatry competencies.

Stages of Psychiatry Residency: Historical Perspective and Current Generalities Regarding Training Patterns

Years 1 and 2

Psychiatry residency training is developmental: residents gradually receive more independence in their learning and supervision. Much of the first 2 years of the 4-year course of study has traditionally been hospital based, involving some of the sickest patients but with more on-site, intensive supervision. During the first year of residency, 6 months' study in medicine and neurology is required. With 9 months of required training on general psychiatric wards and on-call psychiatric emergency services and in substance abuse training and consultation-liaison psychiatry, the first 2 years of residency training is often focused on acutely ill hospitalized patients.

Although some residency programs have tried to incorporate more outpatient and longitudinal rotations in the first 2 years, it is often very difficult to do so because of other factors such as resident work-hours rules, conforming with license requirements, financial reimbursement for residents' time based on providing care on inpatient hospital services, and the need to supervise residents more closely using hospital attending psychiatrists.

The fact that psychiatry residents spend most of their first 2 years on inpatient units (either psychiatric, medical, or neurologic) means that on a practical basis residents are very engaged in collaborative or split treatment. The inpatient psychiatric ward, for example, is an excellent representation of the collaborative work of nurses, who provide much of the direct medical and sometimes psychotherapeutic management; social workers, who provide psychotherapy as well as discharge planning; primary care physicians, general internists, and specialists, who deliver much of the care related to physical medicine; psychologists, who provide psychotherapy as well as psychological testing; psychiatrists, who are the attending psychiatrist; and the residents, who are junior to the psychiatrists. The psychiatrists provide the medication management; other medical services such as electroconvulsive treatment; and overall leadership, evaluation, diagnosis and discharge, etc.

This model has been quite pervasive historically since the onset of general hospital psychiatry, except that up until the last 15 years much of the psychotherapy in the general hospital had been provided by the psychiatry resident or attending psychiatrist. In the past 15 years or so, the length of stay has decreased dramatically and the criteria for admitting patients to the hospital have become more narrow (acute suicidality, acute psychosis, violence, etc.). The inpatient psychiatry model remains very much a split-treatment or collaborative model, but the resident and attending psychiatrist are providing much less of the psychotherapy to the inpatients than in previous years. The length of stay on the inpatient psychiatric unit has become so short that by necessity there has had to be a better division of labor, forcing the psychiatry resident and attending psychiatrist to provide less face-to-face psychotherapy to patients and more of the medication or other medical management.

The nature of the inpatient psychiatry unit has changed dramatically, and therefore so has the role of the psychiatry resident. Residents must be able to provide both integrated and split treatment to patients who have major and acute psychiatric problems. They must be able to work collaboratively with a number of professionals in nursing, psychology, social work, occupational therapy, and medicine in providing patients with care in a hospital setting and must make determinations for patients to be discharged into settings that will provide outpatient psychiatric care. The psychiatry resident and attending psychiatrist must determine—based on a range of fiscal, geographic, and other factors—whether the patient should be discharged to integrated treatment or to split treatment. With most of the first 2 years of residency taking place in the inpatient setting or the psychiatric emergency service, how is the resident to make such decisions for outpatient care? What are the guiding principles for making such determinations? What are the dependent and independent factors that should be addressed and documented in the decision-making process?

Essentially, although it is often considered important for residents to achieve competence in triaging patients for either split treatment or integrated care once they are in their second or third year of training, when the residents themselves are providing more outpatient care, it is also important for residents to learn the skills of triage in years 1 and 2, when they are working in psychiatric emergency departments and on inpatient units and are making plans for patients to be seen as outpatients.

Years 3 and 4

In many psychiatry programs, the third year of residency training provides the bulk of the continuous outpatient year. Residents are usually assigned to an outpatient clinic for most of the time but also may have to meet requirements in specialty areas—geriatric, child and adolescent, and community mental health—if they did not meet them in previous years or if they decide to make their fourth year part of their child and adolescent residency training. The residents are often very busy during this year with scheduling patients, clinics, supervision, and core didactics. In addition, more and more residents are thinking about subspecialty training in child and adolescent psychiatry, so during the third year these residents are interviewing for child and adolescent psychiatry training programs that start in their fourth year of residency. This makes it very important for the resident and the residency training director to ensure that all year-appropriate requirements and competencies are met by the end of the third year of residency training.

It is during the third year of residency training, often the outpatient year, when the issues of split treatment versus integrated treatment are highlighted. In many residency programs, third-year residents begin the year with a list of patients—handed down by the previous residents—for whom medication, not psychotherapy, needs to be provided. The lists of such patients are often long; many of the patients have not been seen for months; and the diagnoses of these patients have remained the same for years.

In some clinics, an attending psychiatrist will not have seen these medication-management patients for years. The medication-management patients may or may not be seen by therapists for psychotherapy, and the therapists may or may not be within the university system. If the patient is receiving psychotherapy from a therapist within the university system and the resident is seeing the patient for medication management, this would be considered split treatment. If the patient is being seen by a therapist outside the university system, it is still a split-treatment arrangement, but it is complicated for the clinicians because collaboration and communication are much more difficult. If the patient is seen only by the resident for medication, this might be called integrated treatment, although some residents might not view their role as providing psychotherapy. In this book we make the case that every interaction with the patient—including providing medication—is in fact an integrated form of care. This makes the issues even more complex, because we believe that a psychotherapeutic doctor–patient relationship occurs with the prescribing or discussion of medication (Tasman et al. 2000).

During the third year of training, the residents see and engage in integrated and split treatment in various settings involving patients with a wide range of ages and diagnoses (children, the elderly, patients in community mental health settings). Supervision is also quite variable. Faculty members tend to supervise the residents—and the residents' cases—while managing large case loads. This is often difficult to do.

Supervision of long-term psychodynamic psychotherapy, often conducted in private practitioners' offices, focuses on dynamic issues, not historically on medication or split-treatment cases; in the community mental health system, residents rely greatly on case workers and social workers for information on patients' social, occupational, and family supports; and the child psychiatry setting is very much based on a collaborative model, relying on social work and psychology and school input into the care of the child. The same may be said for the geriatric setting, where there is a medical model of collaborative care.

The third year is a very busy year for residents, and the competencies are strongly related to the various types of patients, settings, and systems in which the resident is working. The core lectures often do not focus on issues of integrated versus split treatment but more on psychopharmacology directly or psychotherapy history and techniques. The residents can find themselves quite perplexed and with difficult cases. By the end of the third year, the residents are often eager to give up many of their medication patients and some of their more difficult psychotherapy patients to the incoming third-year residents.

How residents decide which patients to give up is very important and should be a critical matter to be determined with an overall supervisor. The problem is that in many residency programs there is not an overall supervisor who knows about all the residents' cases. The supervision throughout the third year in many residency programs is often fragmented. Logs or casebooks have not traditionally been kept by residents, although keeping such logs has been advocated by residency review committees in other disciplines as well as in psychiatry. The upper limits of the numbers of split-treatment cases or integrated-treatment cases a resident should carry during the third year or fourth year or by the time of graduation have not yet been determined for the discipline of psychiatry.

Some university clinics, for example, recommend that third-year residents try to refer stable patients to their primary care physicians for medication management at the end of the year. There are many reasons for this recommendation: 1) too many patients will be on the list for the incoming third-year residents; 2) in a capitated system it is not economical to see patients more frequently, so the university psychiatry clinic loses money every time residents see such patients; and 3) depending on the insurance carrier, there might not be any reimbursement for residents' time when they see medication-management patients (this is dependent on whether there is an attending supervisor who is also seeing the patient). Interestingly, the question of whether these economic issues should be factors in making decisions about educational issues has not been properly addressed by the discipline of psychiatry. Should a resident necessarily be reimbursed for services, when his or her salary is supposedly paid from other sources? Complex issues such as these provide further evidence of the need to carefully evaluate the competency of residents as they complete this very intensive year of providing split treatment and integrated treatment in various settings.

If there is a general adult year 4, it is a good time to review and consolidate skills in integrated versus split treatment. By then residents have had a good overview of both inpatient and outpatient integrated and split treatment in various settings with patients of all ages and comorbidities. The problem with year 4, however, is that it is not homogeneous from one resident to another and from one program to another. Often residents use the fourth year for electives, research, or sharpening their skills in a particular area. Also, if the resident chooses to enter child and adolescent psychiatry, the fourth year is spent in training for this subspecialty. So the fourth year is somewhat inconsistent, and the resident often chooses rotations that might enable him or her to enter residencies in forensics, geriatrics, etc.

The fourth year has traditionally not been a time when residents are thinking of honing their skills in integrated versus split treatment. Residents are thinking instead about jobs and transition to practice. Many of the higher-paying jobs are ones in which clinicians are required to see many patients for evaluations for medication in a short period of time. Such jobs are in systems of care or clinics where the triage for the evaluation is coming from a social worker or psychologist within the system. In other words, these positions are for the psychiatrist to do a lot of medication evaluations and follow up patients in a split-treatment arrangement. Whether or not the psychiatrist can follow up the patient in an integrated model, it is usually not the preferred arrangement.

Residents in their fourth year are often confronted with choices about whether to take such jobs. Residents are generally carrying large debts from their medical school loans, so high-paying, salaried jobs for this kind of split-treatment work is certainly tantalizing. Whether or not residents translate these job searches by going back and asking for more split-treatment cases within the residency programs has not been well studied. The positions being offered to residents on graduation—whether they are in clinics, closed systems of care, or community mental health centers—often require more skills in split treatment. Ensuring that residents are prepared to safely take on such positions is clearly one of the reasons why improved assessment of competencies and skills is needed.

Summary

The success of residents in learning how to deliver integrated and split treatment relies heavily on the developmental sequence of the residency; the type and quality of supervision provided; the core lecture and other didactic experiences; and the clinical experiences and settings and the numbers of patients with certain types of diagnoses, ages, comorbidities, etc. How do all of these clinical and didactic experiences get integrated so that the resident can see the differences and similarities between split and integrated treatment? Given the historical changes that have had dramatic impacts on inpatient and outpatient care and subspecialty training in the last 15 years, has the general adult residency training kept up with the ability to evaluate skills and competencies in the area of integrated versus split treatment? Are residents in both adult and child psychiatry being adequately prepared for their future jobs?

The scope of this book is focused on assessing competencies of residents in split treatment and integrated treatment, a type of assessment that is in its infancy. This is an evolving process. We hope that the ideas set forth in these pages will serve to move the field to discuss, study, and improve the methods of training residents and assessing their skills and competencies so that they will be better prepared to provide excellent psychotherapeutic and pharmacotherapy care, whether in split or integrated treatment. Throughout the book we offer options for assessing competency to provide guideposts for training directors and psychiatry residents.

References

American Medical Association: ACGME program requirements for residency education in psychiatry, in Graduate Medical Education Directory, 2004–2005. Chicago, IL, American Medical Association, 2004, pp 369–370

American Psychiatric Association: Practice guideline for the treatment of patients with bipolar disorder. Am J Psychiatry 151 (12 suppl):1–36, 1994

American Psychiatric Association: Practice guideline for the treatment of patients with schizophrenia. Am J Psychiatry 154 (4 suppl):1–63, 1997

American Psychiatric Association: American Psychiatric Association Practice Guideline for the Treatment of Patients With Major Depressive Disorder, 2nd Edition. Washington, DC, American Psychiatric Publishing, 2000

Barlow DH, Gorman JM, Shear MK, et al: Cognitive-behavioral therapy, imipramine, or their combination for panic disorder: a randomized controlled trial. JAMA 283:2529–2536, 2000

Clarkin JF, Carpenter D, Hull J, et al: Effects of psychoeducational intervention for married patients with bipolar disorder and their spouses. Psychiatr Serv 49:531–533, 1998

Dewan M: Are psychiatrists cost-effective? An analysis of integrated versus split treatment. Am J Psychiatry 156:324–326, 1999

Dunner DL, Schmaling KB, Hendrickson H, et al: Cognitive therapy versus fluoxetine in the treatment of dysthymic disorder. Depression 4:34–41, 1996

Epstein RM, Hundert EM: Defining and assessing professional competence. JAMA 287:226–235, 2002

Goldman W, McColloch J, Cuffel B, et al: Outpatient utilization patterns of integrated and split psychotherapy and pharmacotherapy for depression. Psychiatr Serv 49:477–482, 1998

Keller MB, McCullogh JP, Klein DN, et al: A comparison of nefazodone, the cognitive behavioral-analysis system of psychotherapy, and their combination for the treatment of chronic depression. N Engl J Med 342:1462–1470, 2000

Lohr KN (ed): Medicare: A Strategy for Quality Assurance, Vol 2. Washington, DC, National Academy Press, 1990

Mavissakalian M: Combined behavioral therapy and pharmacotherapy of agoraphobia. J Psychiatr Res 27 (suppl 1):179–191, 1993

Olfson M, Marcus SC, Pincus HA: Trends in office-based psychiatric practice. Am J Psychiatry 156:451–457, 1999

Olfson M, Marcus SC, Druss B, et al: National trends in the outpatient treatment of depression. JAMA 287:203–209, 2002

Riba MB, Balon R (eds): Psychopharmacology and Psychotherapy: A Collaborative Approach. Washington, DC, American Psychiatric Press, 1999

Tasman A, Riba MB, Silk KR (eds): The Doctor-Patient Relationship in Pharmacotherapy: Improving Treatment Effectiveness. New York, Guilford, 2000

U.S. Department of Health and Human Services: Reducing Tobacco Use: A Report of the Surgeon General. Atlanta, GA, Centers for Disease Control and Prevention, 2000

West JC, Wilk JE, Rae DS, et al: Economic grand rounds: financial disincentives for the provision of psychotherapy. Psychiatr Serv 54:1582–1588, 2003

Part I

Integrated Treatment

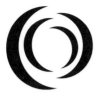

Selection of Medication and Psychotherapy in Integrated Treatment

Thinking About the Issues in Integrated Treatment

Some of the difficulties regarding integrated versus split treatment are related to the following issues: 1) how patients are triaged; 2) who does the evaluation and makes the diagnosis; 3) the experience and skill level of the clinician in various types of psychotherapy; 4) the goals, commitment, and resources of the patient; and 5) what the clinician(s) can hope to reasonably accomplish. Whether the patient is recommended for integrated treatment or split treatment, questions about the type of psychotherapy and the use of medication (whether or not to use it, when to administer it, and what type to use) are clearly relevant factors. In this chapter, we discuss the provision of medication and psychotherapy in an integrated model: the psychiatry resident is providing both the psychotherapy and the medication management or other medical care.

When the Patients Calls for an Appointment

When a patient calls for an appointment to be seen, he or she is having a problem. The patient may have some expectation or view about what he or she might need based on his or her history, the experiences of his or her friends or family members with similar (or different) problems, portrayals in the media, or something that was said by another clinician if a clinician recommended that the patient make the call. Or perhaps the patient has no expectations and just wants help.

As described by Bender and Messner (2003, p. 9), the initial call may be challenging for the novice therapist and also for the patient. It should be approached with the patient's privacy and concerns in mind (Bender and Messner 2003, p. 9). The focus of the initial call is usually scheduling of the initial session and whether insurance will cover costs. A realistic time frame for the initial session should be provided (the time should be suitable for both the patient and the resident without the necessity of rushing in and out), and the length and cost of the session should be specified.

The first moments of the session are very important and could certainly be anxiety provoking for the patient (and also for the resident). The patient may analyze the way he or she is greeted (addressing the patient in the waiting area should be done in a way to preserve the patient's confidentiality), how the resident looks (the resident's facial expression and dress), whether and how the resident shakes the patient's hand, and how the waiting room and office are decorated (whether there are any personal items in the office, etc.). First impressions count in almost every situation, and this is certainly true in the interaction between the doctor and the patient.

Patients often come in with biases, and it is helpful to understand these as well as patients' belief systems (Carli 1999) regarding medication and psychotherapy. For example, some have had successes with psychotropic medication or other types of medication (e.g., antibiotics) in the past and therefore might be open to thinking about medication. If patients have had adverse drug reactions, allergic reactions, or serious side effects from medications, it would be important to discuss these issues.

Patients may be quite frightened about their symptoms and what they imagine or fear about seeing a psychiatrist. There are many stigmatizing portrayals in movies, television, and other media in which seeing a psychiatrist is represented as a potentially scary event with frightening consequences such as being locked up, being placed in a straitjacket, being immediately administered electroconvulsive therapy, or being put in a diabetic coma. Although most patients would probably not be worried about such things, it certainly would behoove the resident to try to assess these issues and begin to allay the patient's fears and worries.

The doctor–patient relationship begins with the telephone call for the initial appointment, and whoever speaks with the patient to schedule the appointment acts as an extension of the physician (Simon 2004). It is therefore important for that person to ask the patient about what led to making the call for the appointment; how that process went; whether there was any difficulty in getting in to see the resident; and then, as part of the history taking, what beliefs and issues the patient has that will need to be sorted out between the patient and the psychiatry resident.

Questions to consider asking the patient include the following:

1. Why did you decide to see someone?
2. When did you decide to call for an appointment?
3. Whom did you speak to arrange the appointment?
4. Did you have any preconceived ideas about what might happen here?
5. Did you encounter any difficulties in making or getting this appointment?

These are open-ended questions that might help elicit issues, thoughts, and feelings that would be important to understand. If these questions are not asked early on, it is sometimes difficult to go back and retrieve important information.

> **Competency:** The psychiatry resident should be able to demonstrate the ability to ask questions regarding why the patient is being seen for a psychiatric evaluation (potentially medication and psychotherapy).

Thinking Broadly

The initial evaluation between the resident and patient is discussed in Chapter 3, "Evaluation and Opening in Integrated Treatment." What we focus on here is that too often the resident is worried about trying to make the diagnosis in the first session with the patient. It could be that the patient has already received a diagnosis from another clinician. Certainly, after seeing the patient the resident needs to do a dictation and needs to have a diagnosis (not only for billing purposes but to review with the supervisor).

But from the patient's point of view, the objective of the first session is often to establish comfort with and trust in the resident. The patient wants to know if the resident has the ability, empathy, skill, and experience to be able to help with his or her presenting symptoms and any future symptoms. Does this resident understand what has brought the patient in to the clinic? Does the resident seem interested in the patient? And if there is some feeling that the resident does understand, what is the hook or draw that will bring the patient back to be seen for follow-up?

The first session between the patient and the resident is critically important because the resident must demonstrate his or her ability to take care of the patient. The patient may or may not have expectations of what the resident is supposed to do or will be doing. The resident must have the skills not only to grasp what is going on the room during the initial session but also to impart a sense of confidence without overwhelming the patient, to provide a focus for future sessions, and to give the patient a reason why he or she should return. This is a lot of work and takes a lot of skill.

The questions that the patient asks during the initial session may be about psychotherapy: Will a couch be used? Will the patient be hypnotized or hospitalized? Will the patient's spouse be asked to join in the sessions? How much will the patient be asked to reveal? How often will the patient need to come to sessions, and for how long—months or years? What is the resident's availability, and will the patient even be seeing the resident for follow-up? The questions may be about medication: Will the patient be forced to take medication? Will it be something like what the patient's sibling or friend has taken? What are the side effects? Will the medication have an impact on sexuality? How long will the patient need to take the medication? How much will it cost?

Often, especially during training years 1–3, the resident may be nervous about the evaluation as well. It is very difficult to make an assessment or diagnosis, decide on some sort of treatment plan, make an alliance with the patient, and feel that there are enough "hooks" that the patient will return for a follow-up appointment. Added to these tasks are decisions that the resident must make regarding the type of psychotherapy that the patient might benefit from, the skill level that the resident possesses to perform the needed psychotherapy, and whether or not medication needs to be discussed and prescribed at the initial interview.

During the initial interview, the resident is engaged in psychotherapy: beginning the doctor–patient relationship; setting an alliance with the patient; learning to understand the resources, coping mechanisms, strengths, and weaknesses of the patient; and setting an agenda for future sessions. Whether the focus of this session is on medication, diagnosis, or other issues, the resident must show competence, confidence, and ability to gauge the patient's capacity for self-reflection and goal setting and must determine whether or not the patient is ready for the next steps. The patient's safety must always be assessed and evaluated. Although the first session should start with open-ended questions, the time restriction will not allow for the entire session to be open ended, so the resident needs to become more directive. The note writing should not be extensive and should be explained to the patient in a positive fashion.

These are very difficult concepts for the resident to master. If the resident is to talk about medication, a diagnosis needs to have been made. For example, one cannot talk about prescribing an antidepressant medication without talking with the patient about a mood disorder. So the resident needs to determine whether the patient is ready to listen to and accept this type of discussion. Similarly, if there is a mood disorder and interpersonal psychotherapy would also be part of the treatment, the resident needs to decide whether to discuss what this type of psychotherapy entails, how many visits are required, the goals of treatment, and how the psychotherapy relates to also taking medication. The resident also needs to find a way to gauge the patient's ability for change (Beitman et al. 2003). Furthermore, if there is a comorbid personality disorder, it needs to be assessed and factored into the treatment plan. Without a good history, it is almost impossible to diagnose a personality disorder.

To summarize, the key ingredients in this first session regarding combined psychotherapy and medication include the following:

1. Forging a doctor–patient alliance
2. Inquiring about how the patient got to the first session
3. Asking about and listening to belief systems about medication and psychotherapy
4. Assessing the patient's capacity for discussion of the diagnosis, treatment plan, and types of therapy
5. Assessing the resident's own capacity to deliver the recommended type of treatment
6. Reassuring the patient about the confidential nature of the treatment but also discussing reasons why the confidentiality might be broken (posing a danger to oneself, posing a danger to others, engaging in child abuse, etc.).

Medication: General Issues to Be Addressed

If medication is one of the treatments that may be of benefit to the patient, the resident must determine and address the following:

1. Is the patient motivated to use medication? If not, what are the factors? Denial? Externalization? (Tasman et al. 2000, p. 93)
2. Which are the target symptoms for the medication? Which ones are most distressing or important to the patient?

3. What are the comorbid medical or other diagnoses that might interact or relate to the use of psychotropic medication?
4. Which side effects of the medication might be most distressing to the patient? To the patient's family members?
5. What might be the obstacles to taking the medication? For example, scheduling of doses; the need for blood assays and laboratory visits; general problems with adherence to taking daily medication; difficulty swallowing; difficulty remembering to take medications; costs of medication; problems with work- or school-related functions (e.g., driving).
6. What beliefs does the patient have about the medication? Does the patient believe that psychotropic medication is addictive or causes brain damage?

The resident needs to provide a fair amount of education to the patient (and possibly to family members) when medication is prescribed. In some states, consent forms for administering medications must be signed by patients, and fact sheets about the medication and side effects must be provided and noted in the chart. These matters all take time, and the resident must gauge how much time there is in the session and decide how much time to use for all of these issues.

Patients and families cannot be hurried. As an example, it might be wise for the resident to begin the discussion of medication but to delay the actual prescribing of medication until the next visit. Information on the medication could be sent home with the patient, as well as information on the diagnosis (e.g., depression). Some patients might also benefit from being informed of good Web sites where additional information might be gleaned. Residents might want to be prepared to direct patients to such Internet sites (Hsiung 2002).

Factors That Affect the Prescribing of Medication

Most importantly, residents need to assess their working alliance with each patient to make the use of medications and psychotherapy successful. In addition, there are skill sets that are important considerations. For the residents, the setting—inpatient versus outpatient—is an important factor.

Inpatient

In the inpatient setting, starting medications is easier for several reasons: the patient can be watched continuously for side effects; the medication is provided by a nurse on a regular schedule; and the cost of the medication is factored into the hospital stay. Often there are groups for discussing medications; many patients are taking medication, so individual patients do not feel singled out; and because patients are not in their usual environment (e.g., home, the workplace), certain issues do not arise such as the need to drive or to have quick reflexes. There are attending psychiatrists, nurses, and other professionals who can speak with the patient and the family to reinforce the diagnosis and the need for medication with certain types of disorders.

Residents are also very well supervised on inpatient units. The attending physician often makes suggestions as to the class, type, and dosage of medication to be used. Inpatient units often tend to use certain types of medication for sleep, anxiety, new-onset psychosis, depression, etc. There are certain prescribing patterns based on hospital formularies and what the attending physicians feel most comfortable with, based on their experiences and the types of patients usually treated in that setting. Residents tend to learn these basic medications, become comfortable prescribing them, and then build on this knowledge base.

On inpatient units, sleep patterns are monitored; appetite changes are evaluated by daily weighing and by noting food remaining on trays; and gastrointestinal side effects are noted. Medications tend to be given in somewhat higher dosages than in the outpatient setting because the dosages can be readjusted quickly. Residents are usually more confident about medication in the hospital setting because there are more professionals around to help the patient deal with the side effects and to provide education and support.

In addition, residents can arrange consultations with other physicians should there be worries about interactions with patients' other medical problems. Family meetings are usually organized to discuss a range of issues, and medications can be an item for discussion if the family and patient so choose. In addition, the hospital usually has medications available in a wide range of preparations (e.g., pills, liquid, and injection), so there are options if the patient has difficulty with one type of preparation. The pharmacists in the hospital are usually very helpful with cutting pills and making it as easy as possible for patients to receive medications that are ordered.

Outpatient

The outpatient setting is more difficult for the resident with regard to prescribing medications. For residents, the most significant difference between inpatient and outpatient settings is that the supervision is usually less intense. In many outpatient settings, there is an attending psychiatrist who sits in for key portions of the initial evaluation of the patient and may discuss initial impressions regarding medication. After this first session, however, the patient may often be seen only by the resident. The attending psychiatrist who first saw the patient may continue to supervise the case. Alternatively, depending on the form of psychotherapy provided to the patient (e.g., cognitive-behavioral therapy), the case might be supervised by someone who is well trained in that type of therapy. The primary supervision, then, might be provided not by a psychiatrist but by a behavioral psychologist. Supervision of the type of medication might be done by a general supervisor, who may be supervising the resident on a number of patients. The resident might discuss only problem cases with the supervisor or might go over every case for a short amount of time. The resident may be quite independent about the type of medication chosen for patients and only bring up particular issues with the supervisor.

As opposed to inpatient units, where there is a steady and constant monitoring of medication issues, there is usually an interval of time between when the patient is first prescribed the medication and when the resident next sees the patient. The resident must inquire about the patient's form of payment for medication to make sure, for example, that the proposed medication will be on the patient's pharmacy formulary. Copayments are an issue, especially for many patients who are taking a number of medications. This is also a matter for discussion.

The resident might want to ask the patient to call and discuss how he or she is doing with the medication before the next appointment, especially if the follow-up appointment is not for a few weeks. The practice of scheduling a follow-up appointment for a new patient several weeks after the initial meeting should be discouraged—the patient should be seen frequently (e.g., within 1 or 2 weeks) during the initial phase of any treatment to help dispel anxieties about the treatment, side effects, and other issues and to foster the doctor–patient relationship. This approach to scheduling helps the resident find out about any negative side effects or problems that the patient might be having with the medication; allows the resident to discuss the dosage (and change it if necessary); and most importantly, enables the patient to feel that the resident cares about the impact of the medication and that the resident and the patient are in a partnership regarding medication.

Some patients want to use e-mail to communicate with the resident, but we urge that communication regarding medication be conducted over the telephone and that such conversations be documented in the patient's chart. There are various problems with e-mail communication (e.g., confidentiality, lack of nonverbal cues), and because there are so many potential problems with medication, we suggest that the telephone be used rather than e-mail (Yager 2003).

Because patients are usually working or are engaged in relationships in the outpatient setting, it is important to find out the impact of taking medications on the job. For example, if the patient is driving as part of his or her job, does the psychotropic medication affect the patient's ability to drive or to have quick reflexes? If so, there may be a need to modify either the medication or the time of day it is taken or to try to have the patient's work responsibilities changed.

Most psychotropic medications affect libido or other sexual side effects, so it is important for the resident to ask the patient questions about these effects. Patients are often too embarrassed to raise such issues and feel more secure when the resident is asking about such important matters. The same is true for weight gain, sleep problems, and constipation, so these must all be routine questions.

Sometimes patients will note that their significant other or various family members are concerned about the medication they are taking. It is helpful for the resident to understand this concern, because it could be a deterrent to the patient's adhering to the medication regimen. It could be useful, for example, to have the concerned family member attend part of a session or a full session with the patient to discuss any problems.

Medication should be kept from young children. It is important for the resident to ascertain who at home might have access to the patient's medication and to make sure that the medication is kept in a safe and secure location. If the patient does not want the children to know about the psychiatric problems or the medication, the resident should discuss this matter with the patient.

At the time of this writing, there is quite a lot of concern about whether antidepressants themselves contribute to suicidality. Data regarding negative or unpublished pharmaceutical trials about this potential problem are being reviewed, and it is hoped that more will be learned. It is important to ascertain the patient's suicidality, homicidality, and potential for violence at every session, particularly when the patient is taking psychotropic medication.

Comorbid Medical Conditions and Substance Abuse/Dependence

Medical Conditions

Residents must be knowledgeable about their patients' medical conditions, what medications their patients are taking, and their patients' medical and surgical histories. Allergies to medications must be noted. Especially in the outpatient setting, the resident must let the patient know that changes in medical condition or medications during the interval between appointments need to be reported to the resident.

Communication between the resident and the primary care providers or specialists needs to be done with the patient's written consent. It is imperative that residents let the other providers know when psychotropic medications are added or changed, again with the patient's written approval. Most patients are very appreciative that such communication occurs. Some patients will be embarrassed or say they will feel stigmatized if their primary care provider or other doctors know about their need for psychotropic medication. In such cases there needs to be frank and open discussion between the resident and the patient, and the resident should point out that he or she cannot provide good care to the patient if such information is not provided to the other clinicians. Serious harm to the patient could result if the other clinicians do not know about the patient's use of psychotropic medication. For example, there could be problems with interactions between medications; changes in blood concentrations of medications could occur if the various prescribers do not know of all the medications the patient is taking. If patients prohibit such communication, the resident must seriously question whether proper care can be provided to the patient, and alternatives must be discussed.

The patient (and all physician and clinician providers) should be clear about who is in charge of what medications. Primary care physicians should not, for example, prescribe psychotropic medication or change dosages without letting the psychiatrist and other mental health clinicians know, and vice versa: the psychiatrist should not prescribe medications other than psychotropic medications (although there are emergency exceptions for both parties). If there is no electronic medical record or if the patient is not being seen in a closed system, the caregivers should discuss ahead of time how to transmit such information in a timely fashion (telephone, e-mail, fax, letter, etc.). It should not be the responsibility of the patient to be the provider of such information.

Substance Abuse/Dependence

Substance abuse and dependence are the subject of another important discussion, especially in the outpatient setting, where patients have greater access to such substances. Patients often do not like to admit their dependence and use of such substances as nicotine, alcohol, marijuana, and other drugs. In addition, there are many patients who have dependences on prescribed drugs such as hydrocodone bitartrate (Vicodin) and oxycodone hydrochloride (Tylox). It is important for the resident not to make assumptions about such problems and to ask questions, make proper referrals for substance abuse treatment, and watch carefully if prescriptions for benzodiazepines, for example, are used up too quickly. If patients are not doing as well as one would expect with a certain medication over a certain period of time, the resident should think about whether there may be a confounding substance problem. If patients are asking for medical leave that is not commensurate with the primary psychiatric diagnosis, then one should think about substance abuse. It is important to obtain a good history of these types of problems when starting treatment and the prescribing of psychotropic medication and then to continue to assess for ongoing problems.

It is also important to consider the role and influence of Alcoholics Anonymous (AA). Frequently, AA participants and sponsors (especially the less experienced ones) discourage patients from using psychotropic medications. They may be right about benzodiazepines but quite wrong about antidepressants (which some AA members call brain depressants).

To summarize, the first encounter with the patient is one of the most difficult for the resident, especially in the outpatient setting. There are multiple issues to assess but the key one is the following:

> **Competency:** At the initial outpatient session, the psychiatry resident must demonstrate the ability to establish a doctor–patient relationship and to provide a trusting, warm environment to explore the patient's needs and problems.

The resident must determine, in the first session or two, what diagnosis to give the patient and, following from that, what type of treatment—psychotherapy, pharmacotherapy, both, neither, etc.—would be recommended.

Factors Affecting Psychotherapy Treatment Planning

Developing a formulation—A biopsychosocial formulation is the key to understanding a patient's diagnosis and treatment plan. Many residents have difficulty with such formulations because they fall short on the "psych" part of the assessment. Often this has to do with not asking enough of the right questions during the interview. Furthermore, residents need to learn to develop hunches and offer them to patients as a beginning point for discussion. This is a difficult skill to teach and hone, because it is based on having experience, seeing a lot of patients, and reading case material—ingredients that are not generally available to a beginning resident.

Selecting the psychotherapy modality—It is almost impossible to recommend a certain modality of psychotherapy without having provided it oneself, or having seen a supervisor or attending psychiatrist provide it, or having read about it. This is where supervision is very important, because the attending psychiatrist must step in and make a recommendation for the type of psychotherapy that might best work for the patient. It is a difficult issue for residents to have to recommend a kind of treatment to a patient without having firsthand knowledge that it will work and benefit the patient. This is one of the aspects of medical care and education that makes one want to hurry up and learn everything as soon as possible. Unfortunately, with various forms of psychotherapy, it is difficult for the beginning resident to do. Sometimes acknowledging such issues for residents in supervision is a good first step. Discussion of selecting a psychotherapy modality in a diagnostic conference with supervisors or a similar venue is probably crucial for the resident's selection of a psychotherapy modality.

Formulating the problem list—Although the psychiatric diagnosis is determined by using the DSM, psychiatrists function under the medical model whereby they need to address the patient's issues in terms of a problem summary list. The patient's presenting problems are added to the list that already exists in the patient's file or electronic medical record. For the psychiatry resident, there are issues of confidentiality, privacy, and other matters that must be addressed in all systems of care. Besides that, however, it is sometimes daunting for residents to actually publicly note a problem on a record that other attending physicians of other medical specialties can read. This is something that needs to be addressed by the supervising attending psychiatrists, and it must be reviewed along with the resident's notes, charts, etc. What goes on the problems list and what comes off it are critically important parts of the patient's record.

Prioritizing problems—It is important for residents to first determine the list of problems and then to determine, with the patient's help, how to prioritize and sequence them. This is difficult work because it often means discussing issues that are not necessarily clear to the patient (or to the clinician) at the time. Sometimes it means waiting for further information or insight from other family members; it could mean waiting for a new job, a change in marital structure, or results of medical tests before determining the next steps. It is important for the resident to exercise patience and guidance without intrusiveness or too much directiveness and without moving too far ahead of the patient.

Determining treatment aims—One of the major tasks for the resident and patient is to determine the aims—both pharmacological and psycho-therapeutic—of the treatment. Once established, the aims should be constantly evaluated and reevaluated and may need to be modified or changed. Few assumptions should be made in the process. But this undertaking is challenging for a novice resident, and combining medication and psychotherapy makes it difficult to tease apart cause and effect. Nevertheless, this is a major task to be addressed at every session and constitutes part of the competency skills of the resident.

Outlining the time frame—One of the questions most frequently asked by patients and their families is how long is the process going to take—how long will they need to take medication, and how long and how often do they need to receive psychotherapy? Most importantly, they want to know how soon they will begin to feel better; how long it will take for the symptoms to improve; when they can go back to work; and when they can expect to start doing better at school. These are difficult but key concepts. For the resident to answer "I don't know" could undermine the confidence the patient has in the treatment process. Yet that may be the best answer the resident can give at the time. It is important for residents to learn how to gauge what the patient is able to understand and the patient's level of distress; they also need to learn the best way to explain the diagnosis and treatment plan and ways that the resident and patient can share in the course of care and recovery.

> **Competency:** During the evaluation phase, the psychiatry resident must be able to demonstrate the ability to develop a biopsychosocial formulation of the patient's problems; develop a problem list; and together with the patient develop treatment aims and prioritize the problems.

References

Beitman BD, Blinder BJ, Thase ME, et al: Integrating Psychotherapy and Pharmacotherapy. New York, WW Norton, 2003

Bender S, Messner E: Becoming a Therapist: What Do I Say, and Why? New York, Guilford, 2003

Carli T: The psychologically informed psychopharmacologist, in Psychopharmacology and Psychotherapy: A Collaborative Approach. Edited by Riba MB, Balon R. Washington, DC, American Psychiatric Press, 1999, pp 179–196

Hsiung RC (ed): E-Therapy: Case Studies, Guiding Principles, and the Clinical Potential of the Internet. New York, WW Norton, 2002

Simon R: Unilateral treatment termination: "You're fired." Psychiatric Times, July 2004, pp 25–26

Tasman A, Riba M, Silk K (eds): The Doctor-Patient Relationship in Pharmacotherapy: Improving Treatment Effectiveness. New York, Guilford, 2000

Yager J: Suggested guidelines for e-mail communication in psychiatric practice. J Clin Psychiatry 64:799–806, 2003

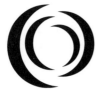

3

Evaluation and Opening in Integrated Treatment

As discussed in Chapter 2, "Selection of Medication and Psychotherapy in Integrated Treatment," the evaluation of any patient begins during the initial contact between the patient and the clinician or whoever is representing the clinician (e.g., triage worker). This could be via an intake telephone call, a referral from another physician, etc. The initial evaluation is focused on collecting the data that the clinician considers pertinent for making the diagnosis and deciding about the treatment. However, it should not be forgotten that the initial evaluation is also about forming the therapeutic alliance.

Because this chapter deals with integrated treatment (the resident providing both the psychotherapy and the medication or other medical care), we do not discuss the diagnosis of and decision making about patients who are referred to a psychiatrist for the sole purpose of treatment with medication or other medical treatment (e.g., electroconvulsive therapy).

In this chapter, we discuss evaluation of the patient and opening of the treatment process (psychopharmacology *and* psychotherapy) by a psychiatrist, either with a new patient or with a patient who was referred to the psychiatrist after therapy with a nonphysician therapist did not work out or for whatever other reason.

It is important to note that the latter situation may happen and that integrated treatment is not and should not be applied only in patients seen de novo (i.e., those seen for the first time by anyone). We would like to emphasize that no matter what the situation (a patient who is being seen for the first time by anyone; a patient who has been referred from someone else), the evaluation should be the same—very thorough and detailed. Nothing should be left unexplored just because the information was already obtained by the referral source and provided to the evaluating psychiatrist. The information from the referral source should be probed and rechecked with the patient. Accepting the interpretation of others could be misleading at times. Reinterpretation of clinical data using newly collected information is generally useful and helpful.

It should be made clear during the first contact that the initial session (or possibly a few initial sessions) is going to be devoted to an evaluation, and only after its completion will any decision about treatment modality or modalities ensue.

Bender and Messner (2003) suggest that framing the first session as a consultation and evaluation may have an important advantage. Both the patient and the psychiatrist can evaluate whether they are a good match and whether they feel comfortable working with each other. Both are given "the freedom to view the first meeting as an introduction without an obligation to continue" (Bender and Messner (2003, p. 17). Framing the first contact as a consultation is probably much easier in an outpatient setting. The concept of the first session (or sessions) being a consultation/evaluation may be also very useful in starting the treatment of children or adolescents. There are more parties involved, such as one or both parents, and getting a good match is therefore more complicated.

The initial step in the evaluation for integrated treatment (or any treatment) is establishing an accurate diagnosis. It is important to emphasize that although the diagnosis is an important element in treatment decision making, it is not the sole element. The diagnosis does not provide much information about the individual and about the individual's need and particular issues in treatment planning. There are other elements—such as the patient's previous response to treatment, symptoms (e.g., sleep disturbance, suicidality), cooperation or resistance, family history, support system, medical history, treatment with other medication, possible previous treatment experience, and value and belief system; and the physician's skills—that may have a significant impact on treatment planning. Thus, information about all these and other factors should be gathered in the first session (or sessions) to help inform the decision about treatment.

First Contact: Technical Remarks

The first contact between the psychiatrist and the patient usually starts in the waiting area. After being triaged and being given an appointment, the patient arrives full of various expectations and usually in a state of heightened expectations. The first impression is quite important. The patient is probably wondering, "Who is this doctor? What is he or she going to ask? Are we going to get along?" The patient is probably feeling a bit uncomfortable in the waiting area and does not want anybody else to know that he is coming to see a psychiatrist. In this era of increased concerns about confidentiality, the psychiatrist needs to make sure that the patient's identity is protected. Therefore, calling the patient by his last name in the waiting area might be problematic, because it reveals the patient's identity. The psychiatrist can call the patient by his first name; however, that may not sit well with some patients, especially older patients. Many experts (e.g., Bender and Messner 2003) therefore advise psychiatrists to simply identify the patient who is waiting, approach the patient, ask whether he is waiting to see this particular psychiatrist, and then invite the patient to follow or come in.

After taking the patient to the office and making him as comfortable as possible (the patient might not feel comfortable spending the entire session sitting in his coat and clutching a bag with medication and other materials in his lap), the resident should explain what is going to happen during the first session or two. It should be made clear approximately how long the session is going to last and what is expected to come out of it. One should be aware that this is the time when the formation of the therapeutic alliance begins. As Bender and Messner (2003, p. 29) point out, the therapist should be responsive and not overbearing at this time (and at other times) and should be careful not to underdirect or overdirect the first session.

The resident should be observant of the patient's behavior during this period: does the patient seem anxious, avoid making eye contact, wring his hands, have tremors, or sit at the edge of the chair? It is also polite, appropriate, and practical to inform the patient that confidential notes will be taken during the information-gathering session, if this is the case. The patient's feelings about the psychiatrist's note taking during the session should also be explored. As MacKinnon and Yudofsky (1991, p. 10) note, some patients may resent the psychiatrist taking *no* notes during the interview, because it would make them feel that what they said was not sufficiently important or that the doctor was uninterested. Other patients, as MacKinnon and Yudofsky also noted, cannot tolerate note taking because they feel that it distracts the psychiatrist's attention from them.

It is also important to make sure that writing information down does not become the dominant activity of the information gathering session. One should write the basic information and scribble down the most important data without interrupting the flow of the interview and without avoiding eye contact with the patient. There may also be times during the interview when the interviewer should stop writing notes, putting the pen and paper down. This applies to situations when intimate or sensitive issues, such as sexual issues or negative feelings about any previous treatment and therapist or physician, are discussed (MacKinnon and Yudofsky 1991).

In these times when nearly everything is computerized, many psychiatrists are switching to electronic medical records. The same rules applicable to paper writing apply to typing electronic notes. We advise psychiatrists not to type into the computer during the session (although we have heard of and witnessed nonpsychiatrist physicians doing so). Paper notes could be transferred into the computer after the session. It is also advisable to transcribe or type notes right away after seeing the patient and not wait until the end of a busy day, when the memories of several patient histories could merge and facts could get confused. (We have also witnessed nonpsychiatrist physicians dictating notes in front of patients.)

Many psychiatrists start the initial evaluation by obtaining basic patient data such as age, marital status, and employment. Others advocate beginning the session with an open-ended question such as "Why are you coming to see me?"; "What can I do for you?"; or "How can I help you?" The patient should be left to answer this question without interruption if possible (although manic or psychotic patients may have to be interrupted). The psychiatrist should acknowledge that he or she is listening by occasionally making comments or sounds such as "Hmm" or "Interesting." The patient should be asked to provide more details whenever possible and appropriate. The psychiatrist should encourage the patient by making comments such as "Tell me more about this" whenever necessary. One should also think and frame questions in terms such as "Why now; why at this point in the patient's life is she coming to see me and telling me this?"

Although we discuss the information gathering in a certain structural fashion, progressing from the chief complaint and present illness through various parts of the history to the mental status examination, it is important to realize that 1) there are many overlaps between various parts of the examination (e.g., present illness and parts of the mental status examination); 2) the sequence of the patient evaluation is not engraved in stone; and 3) the resident should not avoid following cues for the sake of keeping to a rigid information-gathering outline. One mistake that is frequently made by beginning clinicians is putting aside certain matters that are seemingly unrelated to the questions asked. This could lead to missing a very important therapeutic issue, and it could also make the patient feel that the resident is not really interested in his or her concerns. An example of a psychiatrist missing a cue is a situation in which a patient responded to the opening question, "What is bringing you here?" by saying, with her eyes full of tears, "I am a widow." The response by the inexperienced resident was, "OK, but why are you here now?"

The initial evaluation is usually finished in a preliminary form within the first hour or so designated for the assessment. Evaluation of an inpatient (but not in the emergency department) may require more time. Often even the most experienced clinician may not be able to finish the initial evaluation and establish a preliminary diagnosis within the time frame of the first contact, and a subsequent evaluation session may have to be scheduled. Most initial evaluations of adult patients include evaluation of the patient himself or herself. The evaluation, however, may involve an interview of relatives or significant others in some cases. An evaluation of a child or adolescent should always, if possible, include an interview of parents or guardians (together with the child and also separately).

Initial Evaluation Outline

It is important to note that the order of various parts of the initial evaluation may be a matter of personal preference or custom. However, after obtaining basic identifying data, one should start with the inquiry about the chief complaint and present illness.

Chief Complaint and Present Illness

Even though the chief complaint is traditionally listed on outlines and forms of psychiatric evaluations, it is not something one always asks about, but rather identifies in the written summary of the examination. It could be a direct quote of the patient's response to the question, "How can I help you?" or "Why do you think you need help?" Or it could be a very brief, simple summary of the patient's main complaint ("Patient has been depressed for the past 3 weeks," or "Sudden onset of panic attacks 3 weeks ago"). It may also serve as an introduction to the next part of the evaluation: the present illness.

The questioning about the history of the present illness should start with open-ended questions. These broad questions, however, should be replaced—depending on the clinical situation—by focused or targeted specific questions about the symptoms, their onset, possible precipitating factors, impact on functioning, the scope of distress, maladaptive patterns, and other issues. Some patients may be able to provide a fairly chronological account of their present illness. Others may need to be asked specific questions about the onset and other clinical factors. Depending on the clinical material provided by the patient, one may ask questions that may later help in the treatment selection (medication, psychotherapy, or both). The questioning usually becomes more direct and targeted through the interview. It may not always be possible to clearly separate the history of the present illness from the past psychiatric history or history of previous psychiatric illnesses. An example is the case of recurrent major depression. The most recent episode of depression may represent the present illness, but one should not totally separate it from previous episodes of depression. The history of the present illness could include what some call the psychiatric review of systems (MacKinnon and Yudofsky 1991). This review includes questions about the patient's sleep pattern, appetite, weight regulation, bowel functioning, and sexual functioning (MacKinnon and Yudofsky 1991). Assessment of suicidality should be also included in this part of the evaluation. Assessment of suicidality could start with broader questions such as asking whether the patient has been feeling that life is not worth living. The assessment of suicidality and homicidality, however, should ultimately be specific and well documented. (Does the patient have vague suicidal ideation or a specific plan? If the patient has a plan, is the selected modality available? What is the overall risk? Is a safety net available?) Some clinics use standardized screening tools and guidelines for suicidality to help with consistency and training of residents (American Psychiatric Association 2003).

The interviewer should not remain focused on only one area of the problem and psychopathology. After establishing a very preliminary possible diagnosis, one should always probe other areas of psychopathology (e.g., in depressed patients one asks about anxiety, psychosis, etc.).

Psychiatric and Medical Illness History

The patient's history of psychiatric illness is a very important part of the initial evaluation. Such a history could have a tremendous impact on treatment planning and selection of treatment modality. A patient with a recent episode of major depression and a history of two previous episodes of major depression should probably start lifelong treatment of this illness. The suicidality of a patient with a history of several serious suicide attempts is going to be viewed much more seriously than a suicidal gesture in a patient with no previous history of suicidality. A positive response to previous treatment should guide one to use the same treatment again and vice versa—an unsuccessful treatment trial should guide one not to use the same modality again.

The patient should be probed about onset, possible precipitating factors, course, comorbidity, accompanying disability, and treatment. As noted above under "Chief Complaint and Present Illness," at times it is difficult to separate the history of the present illness and the overall psychiatric illness history. Information about psychiatric hospitalizations should include the patient's age at the time of hospitalization, reason for hospitalization, length of hospitalization, place of hospitalization (the psychiatrist may be familiar with the place and may need to obtain records from the hospital), what was done during the hospitalization (medications tried, psychotherapy), the patient's condition at discharge, and the patient's feelings about the hospitalization.

The patient should be asked about previously used treatment. Questions about medications should include the names of the medications, the patient's understanding of the reasons for using a particular medication, the length of treatment with each particular medication, maximum dosages, whether the medication was helpful, which symptoms were relieved the most, and what side effects were present. Questions about medication allergies should be also asked, but one should make a distinction between true allergy and a serious side effect. Many psychotic patients will frequently say that they are allergic to one of the antipsychotics. Detailed questioning may reveal that they had a dystonic reaction when taking a higher dosage. The patient should also be asked whether he or she is taking any psychotropic medication at the time of the initial evaluation. As Bender and Messner (2003) emphasize, one should not assume that the patient is not taking psychotropic medication if he or she is not seeing a psychiatrist. Many primary care physicians prescribe psychotropic medications. Many primary care physicians are even mandated by managed care companies to try psychotropic medication and to refer the patient to a psychiatrist only after the first treatment attempt fails. Questions (when, why, what kind, success/failure, patient's feelings about the treatment) should be asked about previous psychotherapy and behavioral therapy. One should also ask whether medication was combined with psychotherapy or behavioral therapy in the past.

Previous suicidal thoughts and behavior should be explored and documented (age at the time of suicide attempt, relationship to symptoms, planned or impulsive attempt, modality used, feelings about death and dying at the time of the suicide attempt, whether it was a suicidal gesture, subsequent treatment, and the patient's current feelings about a particular suicide attempt). It is also important to make a distinction between suicidal and self-mutilatory behavior.

A thorough exploration of possible substance abuse history may be part of the overall psychiatric history or part of the personal and social history. The patient should be asked about substances abused (specific substances could be mentioned), age at commencement of substance abuse, duration (if not continuous), frequency, amount used, money spent for substance abuse, how the substance was obtained, possible association with illegal activities (e.g., selling drugs), complications (medical, e.g., hepatitis, acquired immune deficiency syndrome; psychiatric, e.g., depression, withdrawal, blackouts; relational; financial; employment-related), immediate effect of the substance abused (feeling better, improved mood, relief of anxiety), personal feelings about substance abuse (feelings of guilt or shame), in what situation substance occurs (alone, with a group), previous treatment and its results (inpatient, outpatient). Similar questions should be asked specifically about alcohol abuse. Patients should also be questioned about tobacco (smoking or chewing, and how much) and caffeine use (the number cups of coffee a day, the amount of other caffeinated beverages).

Medical history is an important part of the psychiatric evaluation. The history of serious illnesses, especially chronic ones, and surgeries should be obtained. The resident should consider whether the presenting symptoms are either a manifestation of the chronic illness, a reaction to the chronic illness, or not related to the illness. Specific questions should also be asked to determine the possibility of a seizure disorder or head injury. The patient should also be asked about medications used to treat any medical conditions. Preferably the patient should provide a list of these medications and dosages. Many medications can induce various symptoms—such as depression, anxiety, and fatigue—and thus mimic mental disorders. Many medications can also interfere with the metabolism of psychotropic agents.

Female patients should always be asked about their menstrual history, including the age at menarche, regularity of the cycle, possible menopause depending on age, use of contraceptives, and symptoms associated with menstruation (pain, cramping, changes of mood, irritability), including their possible alleviation with hormones and medications (e.g., antidepressants). Women of childbearing age should be questioned and possibly tested regarding the possibility of pregnancy before starting medication.

The medical history could also include a brief review of systems.

Family History

Information about a family history of psychiatric illness and responses to treatment could also have an impact on treatment selection and planning.

Family history should include the family history of psychiatric and medical illness and exploration of relationships within the family. Information about both parents should include their ages if living (or age at the time of death and cause of death), history of mental disorders, history of medical illnesses, medications used to treat any psychiatric illnesses, and responses to medications. The information about siblings should include their ages (and thus also the patient's birth order), presence of psychiatric illnesses, treatments, and responses to treatments. A history of psychiatric illness and treatment in members of the extended family (grandparents, aunts, uncles, cousins) should also be obtained. Besides asking about mental illness, we recommend asking specifically about substance abuse and suicide history in family members. Many people do not think about substance abuse or suicide in terms of mental illness. One should also explore the relationships within the family: how the patient gets along with his or her parents and siblings, whether there has been any violence within the family, and whether any abuse (physical or sexual) has occurred.

Personal and Social History

Personal and social history is the part of the evaluation that makes the psychiatric evaluation different from an ordinary medical evaluation. Physicians in other disciplines may ask about parts of the personal history but do not usually obtain the personal and social history in its entirety. This part of the evaluation may help the examining physician with treatment planning in terms of the patient's preferences, family and social support, financial situation, affordability of various treatments, and other factors involved in treatment planning. The personal and social history encompasses several areas, and the clinician should attempt to elicit a full picture of the patient and his or her life situation.

The personal history may start with the perinatal and developmental history. Information about the prenatal situation (family constellation, whether the parents wanted and planned to have this child, possible complications of pregnancy) and the patient's birth (premature, uncomplicated, forceps delivery, cesarean section, jaundice at birth, defect at birth, etc.) should be obtained. Many pieces of information that some recommend gathering—such as the parents' reaction to the patient's gender and selection of the patient's name (MacKinnon and Yudofsky 1991)—might not be realistically obtainable under the ever-present time pressure. Some trainees, however, may have the luxury of having enough time to obtain this kind of information. Further information about personal history should include, if time and situation permit, developmental milestones, relationships during childhood and adolescence, and emerging personality (shy, defiant, oppositional) during childhood and adolescence.

Educational history should include information regarding whether the patient graduated from high school (if not, why not and whether a General Educational Development (GED) diploma was obtained), college education, postgraduate education (versus current employment), and original educational plans and their fulfillment. The patient should be asked about any history of difficulties, academic or behavioral, at school.

Occupational history should include, if possible, information about all employment, duration, reason for termination or change, any difficulties at work, and possible exposure to dangerous substances. An important question to consider is whether the patient's employment is commensurate with his or her education level.

Military history should include the age when the patient was drafted or recruited, reasons for signing up (idealism, financial reasons, or risk and thrill seeking), length of service, and the nature of and reason for discharge. It should also include information about whether the patient experienced combat, sustained any injuries, underwent any disciplinary actions, and was exposed to substances of abuse during service.

Relational and marital history should include information about any sustained relationship in the patient's life. Inquiry should be made about the age when the patient got married, length of marriage or relationship, past conflicts and disagreements, and present relationship with the partner or spouse. If the patient is divorced, reasons for divorce should be discussed. Information about children—their ages, health, education, and patient's relationship with them—should also be gathered. When the patient presents relational or marital issues as the core of his or her problems, the relational and marital history can be expanded by asking about further issues such as areas of disagreement, who does what at home, management of family finances, and relationships with members of the extended family.

Sexual history should include information about psychosexual development, early sexuality, sexual orientation, age of first sexual contact or intercourse, frequency of sexual activity, ability to reach orgasm, any sexual dysfunction (low libido, erectile dysfunction, lack of lubrication, premature ejaculation, delayed orgasm, anorgasmia, painful orgasm), masturbation, and unusual sexual preferences. We have noted that psychiatric residents frequently omit the sexual history for various reasons, either being uncomfortable asking patients about sex or inappropriately worrying about offending patients by asking about sexual history. We would like to emphasize that when asked tactfully and in full confidentiality, patients do not usually feel offended by questions about their sexuality, and in fact appreciate that someone is taking the time to ask about this often-neglected subject.

Some (e.g., MacKinnon and Yudofsky 1991) also suggest asking about social relationships, friends, religious and cultural background, hobbies, and long-term plans as a part of personal history. Others (e.g., Bender and Messner 2003, p. 66) recommend obtaining an "adaptive history" by asking questions such as "What stresses have you overcome in the past?"; "How did you do it?"; "What are your personal strengths?"; and others.

Mental Status Examination

The mental status examination is a summary of the physician's observation and the patient's subjective reporting of various areas such as appearance, behavior, feelings, perception, thinking, and cognitive functioning. Most textbooks describe the mental status examination as a long list of categories to be examined at the end of the psychiatric evaluation. An experienced clinician, however, usually begins the mental status examination from the very beginning of the evaluation by observing the patient's appearance and behavior and registering symptoms the patient reports. The more formal mental status examination conducted at the end of the psychiatric evaluation should therefore address only areas not previously covered, or areas in need of further clarification. One should not repeat detailed questioning about all symptoms of major depression in a patient who presented with a chief complaint of depressed mood, low energy, poor sleep, and lack of appetite. One might, however, ask about symptoms not mentioned before, such as anhedonia or cognitive impairment.

The mental status examination should include but not be limited to the following areas:

Attitude—Whether the patient comes into the office voluntarily or hesitantly; whether the patient is cooperative, friendly, and appropriate; whether he or she makes good or poor eye contact; and the nature of the patient's facial expression.

Appearance—The patient's hygiene, clothing, and special marks (e.g., tattoos).

Behavior and psychomotor activity—The nature of the patient's gait; whether he or she is restless, sits on the edge of the chair, is wringing the hands, has increased motor activity; whether the patient has abnormal movements, tics, dystonias, gesticulations, etc.

Speech—The quantity (e.g., talking all the time or answering only in monosyllabic words) and quality (errors, tone, rate of production, rhythm, etc.) of the patient's speech.

Affect, mood, and their appropriateness and stability (vs. lability)—The "vegetative" signs such as sleep (including dreams), appetite, and libido should also be explored. Exploration of this area should also include other symptoms of mood disorders such as possible anhedonia, energy level, and feelings of guilt. Finally, one should ask about recent suicidal or homicidal ideation and possible plans.

Anxiety and related symptoms—Obsessions, compulsions, panic attacks, social avoidance, phobias, flashbacks, and startled responses.

Perception—Illusions, hallucinations, and feelings of unreality and depersonalization.

Thinking—Form (e.g., flow of associations, blocking, tangentiality, circumstantiality) and content (e.g., suspiciousness, ideas of reference, thought insertion, delusions—systematized, vague, or isolated—and their content—paranoid or grandiose) of the patient's thought processes; also, in the case of mood disorders, congruency with mood.

Alertness and wakefulness.

Orientation—By time, place, person, and situation.

Concentration—Tested by simple tasks such as serial sevens or spelling certain words forward and backward.

Memory—Recent, intermediate, remote, possible confabulation. Short-term memory and concentration could be tested by asking the patient to remember three things and asking him or her to recall them in 5 minutes.

Estimate of general information and fund of knowledge—The patient's ability to provide information about recent events, big cities, famous people, or geography.

Estimate of intelligence—Average, below average, above average, or possible mental retardation.

Judgment—Operational and formal; estimated by asking about reactions to standard situations.

Abstraction—The patient's ability to abstract could be tested by asking him or her to interpret proverbs or by discussing similarities and differences.

Insight—The patient's awareness of his or her illness or situation.

Impulse control and frustration tolerance.

Formulation

After finishing the evaluation, the examining resident may briefly formulate the case for himself or herself, considering the key issues such as the patient's present illness, past and personal history, developmental issues, and ego strengths and defenses. The formulation, however, may be postponed until further information is gathered and any test results have been obtained.

Diagnosis

Diagnosis (or diagnoses) of the patient should be made using the multiaxial DSM diagnostic classification (American Psychiatric Association 2000). Many consider the multiaxial diagnosis cumbersome and insufficiently inclusive. However, it forces the clinician to consider various areas that may have an impact on treatment planning and treatment outcome: diagnosis of major mental disorder, possible personality disorder or its traits, intellectual impairment, the presence of physical illness possibly involved in the pathogenesis and possibly complicating the treatment planning and outcome, the presence of major stressors, and the level of functioning.

Diagnostic considerations might include decisions about further areas of possible exploration such as a physical examination, laboratory testing (either exploratory, such as thyroid testing in unexplained tiredness and low energy, or as a baseline before starting certain medications, such as liver enzyme testing before beginning certain antipsychotics; or blood urea nitrogen, creatinine, and thyroid tests before starting lithium), measurement of heart rate and blood pressure before starting some medications, ordering possible psychological testing (e.g., memory and other cognitive testing), and ordering neurological examination and other specialized diagnostic testing.

> **Competency:** The psychiatry resident should, based on his or her evaluation of the patient, be able to select the appropriate combination of pharmacotherapy and psychotherapy.

Treatment Planning

The entire initial evaluation is focused on establishing the diagnosis and selecting the most appropriate treatment. Both the diagnosis and the treatment selection and plan should be thoroughly discussed with the patient at the end of the initial evaluation (see "Discussion With the Patient/Opening" below). The treatment selection is a very complicated process, which includes (in no particular order of importance and not exclusively) diagnosis; comorbidity; the evidence-based medicine data; possible use of guidelines; consideration of target symptoms; previous treatment experience (both efficacy and side effects); dangerousness (suicidality); the patient's beliefs, possible illness denial, preferences, misconceptions, and expectations; the patient's level of functioning and impairment; the patient's personality traits or personality disorder; possible nonadherence to the medication regimen; possible involvement of another specialist (e.g., a nutritionist in the case of an eating disorder); psychodynamic issues; consideration of possible side effects; the physician's experience and skills; formation of the therapeutic alliance; cost of treatment; insurance regulations; availability of both patient and treating physician; physical location of treatment (inpatient, day treatment, outpatient); existence of a support network; and also market seductions and pressures (on both physician and patient, such as those produced by direct consumer advertisement).

Bender and Messner (2003) suggest organizing psychiatric diagnoses into two categories: 1) disorders with targetable symptoms that meet DSM diagnostic criteria (e.g., mood disorders, anxiety disorders, substance abuse), and 2) conditions more closely linked to ongoing life stressors (relational problems, occupational problems, adjustment disorders, personality disorders). This distinction may seemingly help to make the decision about medication versus psychotherapy. Psychotherapy, however, is usually indicated in both categories, and medication could be indicated in either category or both categories. In many instances, the impairment of daily functioning may be a major factor in choosing medication. For instance, the physician may recommend starting cognitive-behavioral therapy in a case of major depressive disorder with mild or no functional impairment; however, he or she will recommend an antidepressant plus cognitive-behavioral therapy in the case of major depressive disorder with severe functional impairment. The decision about selecting psychotherapy could be either therapist-based (whatever psychotherapy is the therapist's area of expertise), diagnosis-based (cognitive-behavioral therapy for depression or in vivo desensitization for agoraphobia without a history of panic attacks), or outcome-based (whatever the goal of therapy is, whatever could be realistically achieved; Makover 2004). Assuming that the evaluating psychiatry resident is competent in various psychotherapies, the decision making at the beginning of integrated treatment is going to a diagnosis-based and outcome-based approach. Let us take a case of major depressive disorder. After considering numerous factors and selecting the most appropriate antidepressant, the psychiatrist may consider the diagnosis and immediate goals in selecting cognitive-behavioral therapy.

> **Competency:** The psychiatry resident should be able to discuss with and explain to the patient the selection of treatment modalities and their rationale.

Discussion With the Patient/Opening

Discussing the diagnosis and the treatment selection and plan with the patient is usually the last step of the initial evaluation (unless the evaluation needs to be extended beyond the first session).

The patient should be informed, in simple terms, regarding the diagnosis and what the diagnosis means in practical terms. He should be encouraged to ask questions about the diagnosis and the diagnostic process. Interestingly, many patients are quite relieved once the diagnosis is made and they have a term—a symbolic explanation—for their problems.

After discussing the diagnosis, the resident should briefly outline the initial treatment plan. The resident should explain the selection of both the medication and psychotherapy, what to expect of each modality, the time frame (e.g., fairly quick alleviation of anxiety with benzodiazepines vs. 3 weeks waiting for an antidepressant to alleviate depressed mood), and possible side effects and their management. The patient should be also given instructions on how to reach the resident in case there is an emergency or if the patient experiences any bothersome side effects or has any questions. Patients especially appreciate the possibility of such contact, and the availability of the resident often alleviates a lot of their anxiety about starting treatment. As with the diagnosis, patients should be encouraged to ask questions about the treatment. Many patients may have very specific questions based on their Internet searches, direct consumer advertisement, or media reports or sensationalism. Finally, the patient should be given a follow-up appointment fairly soon (it is simply not acceptable to say, "Here is your prescription; see me in month or two"). Patients should be seen fairly frequently during the initial phase of any treatment.

As Beitman and colleagues (2003, p. 38) explain, the initiation of treatment should also include summarizing the patient's conceptualization of the illness and expectations of treatment, predicting possible side effects of pharmacotherapy, acknowledging negative treatment experiences, addressing the patient's denial of illness or need for treatment with inquiry into negative social consequences or lifestyle, and, in the case of pharmacotherapy, comparing mental illness and psychopharmacology to other medical problems and drugs such as diabetes and insulin.

The subsequent sessions during the opening phase of treatment may further deal with issues such as the meaning of medication, fear of addiction to medication, loss of control over behavior, loss of personality, confusion of symptoms and side effects, the natural tendency to stop treatment when symptoms improve, and benefits and drawbacks of treatment (Beitman et al. 2003).

Pruett and Martin (2003) suggest other issues one should be aware of when prescribing medication and combining it with psychotherapy, such as the following:

- The clinician should be constantly aware of the seductions of marketing.
- Psychodynamic formulations are not a luxury but are necessary for making good treatment choices and for evaluating and reevaluating (on an ongoing basis) drug choice and the effectiveness of combined treatment.
- Psychiatrists should not be intimidated by time pressures, especially in the early appointments.
- Discussions of chemical imbalances are generally less helpful than many clinicians think, because it is so difficult to predict what they will mean to any given patient.
- The clinician should neither oversell nor undersell any one drug as a part of the treatment regimen but should instead tell the patient that there are other choices.
- **Psychiatrists should treat their patients as though the therapeutic relationship matters more than the pills—because it usually does.**

Once the initial evaluation—in one or more sessions—is completed, all information is gathered, and various treatment issues mentioned in this chapter are considered, the trainee should discuss the case with the clinical supervisor. The discussion of the diagnosis should include consideration of the impact of the diagnosis on treatment selection and, in the case of integrated or combined treatment, on the sequencing of treatment modalities.

Once the psychiatrist decides to initiate integrated treatment, he or she has to decide about sequencing pharmacotherapy and psychotherapy (which one to start first, or start both at the same time). Sequencing of integrated treatment is discussed in Chapter 4, "Sequencing in Integrated Treatment."

References

American Psychiatric Association: Diagnostic and Statistical Manual of Mental Disorders, 4th Edition, Text Revision. Washington, DC, American Psychiatric Association, 2000

American Psychiatric Association: Practice guideline for the assessment and treatment of patients with suicidal behaviors. Am J Psychiatry 160 (11 suppl):1–60, 2003

Beitman BD, Blinder BJ, Thase ME, et al: Integrating Psychotherapy and Pharmacotherapy: Dissolving the Mind-Brain Barrier. New York, WW Norton, 2003

Bender S, Messner E: Becoming a Therapist: What Do I Say, and Why? New York, Guilford, 2003

MacKinnon RA, Yudofsky SC: Principles of the Psychiatric Evaluation. Philadelphia, PA, JB Lippincott, 1991

Makover RB: Treatment Planning for Psychotherapists: A Practical Guide to Better Outcomes, 2nd Edition. Arlington, VA, American Psychiatric Publishing, 2004

Pruett KD, Martin A: Thinking about prescribing: the psychology of psychopharmacology, in Pediatric Psychopharmacology: Principles and Practice. Edited by Martin A, Scahill L, Charney DS, et al. New York, Oxford University Press, 2003, pp 417–425

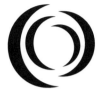

Sequencing in Integrated Treatment

$\mathbf{O}$ne of the most difficult issues for any psychiatrist—either a seasoned clinician or a junior resident—is to determine a treatment plan based on a good working diagnosis. Developing a treatment plan that the patient can reasonably adhere to, that is based on realistic expectations for treating the patient's illness in a timely manner, and that is financially affordable for the patient is surely the goal. Some would say, however, that this is a combination of art and science. Some might argue that the development of treatment plans should be protocol or guideline driven. Others might counter that there are so many factors to be weighed in a realistic treatment plan that it would be difficult to regulate something that is so individualistically driven.

Residents will probably combine medication with various therapy modalities, with supportive and cognitive-behavioral treatment probably being the most frequently used ones. The combination of antidepressant medication and cognitive-behavioral therapy (CBT) has emerged as one of the most effective and beneficial treatment approaches for individuals with chronic mood disorders (Dunner 2001). For instance, the combination of nefazodone and CBT was significantly more efficacious than either treatment alone (Keller et al. 2000), and the combination of these two treatment modalities provided greater psychosocial improvement (Hirschfeld et al. 2002). Although there have been some systematic studies to date of the combination of medication with psychodynamic psychotherapies (Burnand et al. 2002; de Jonghe et al. 2001), it still remains difficult to determine which one is most effective for a particular patient. Furthermore, most of the current studies are trying to compare psychodynamic treatments to medication rather than assessing possible synergistic benefits of the combination of psychotherapy and pharmacotherapy (Roose 2001).

Yet there need to be guideposts for the training of residents. Psychiatry residents must be provided with the framework to think through the various issues to be considered in prescribing psychotropic medication as well as providing psychotherapy as part of integrated treatment.

Once a working diagnosis is developed, the resident must think through a series of issues related to medication and psychotherapy. In this chapter, we explore the various dimensions of this relationship between medication and psychotherapy to provide a practical framework. Without much systematic data, we are left to use clinical experiences as a major basis for recommendations.

Sequence

Let us begin by saying that the diagnosis very much matters. There has historically been a dualism in psychiatry as shown by the Axis I–Axis II dichotomy, with a split regarding dynamic theories and medication. Many psychoanalysts, for example, view medication as an adjunct to the dynamic theory and as a recourse to be used only if the dynamic treatment is not sufficient. At the other end of the spectrum are primary care physicians or very biologically oriented psychiatrists who use psychotropic medication and then make a referral to a mental health professional for psychotherapy if the patient is not improving with the medication.

Furthermore, Axis III diagnoses are also critically important. One needs to understand what medications the patient is currently taking; the patient's past and present medical history; the patient's family medical history; the patient's allergies; and any other symptoms that might be related to an underlying medical condition. If a patient has not been seen by his or her primary care physician or other physician for quite a while, it might be a good idea to suggest a checkup. If the patient has current and complicated medical problems, it might be a good idea for the psychiatry resident to receive permission to call the primary care physician to discuss the patient's current medical condition and to inquire whether the physician has any thoughts about the treatment plan for the psychiatric problems.

The resident will want to know the patient's weight, height, and vital signs (including blood pressure) at the initiation of any type of treatment. These indices may be regularly checked by the clinic or ordered by the resident at the first visit and at intervals thereafter. The resident should also have access to any recent laboratory reports on the patient that might be helpful, such as blood sugar, liver enzymes, and thyroid functions.

The approach used in most of medicine is to try one treatment first and see if it works. Combinations of medications are prescribed, but they usually do not start off as combinations. Instead they are sequenced. This is done so that the clinician can observe the effectiveness of one; see if there are any untoward effects, such as an allergic reaction; and determine whether the medication is causing other side effects such as a sexual side effect, jitteriness, etc. When psychiatrists used to prescribe powerful antipsychotic medications with antidopaminergic and anticholinergic effects (e.g., thioridazine, chlorpromazine, and haloperidol), there was a strong focus on treating the side effects early to keep the patient comfortable and to ensure adherence to the medication regimen. There was also the desire to make sure that these medications did not mask symptoms of tardive dyskinesia, which could become irreversible. So the tradition was to start with one medication and then add others to help augment the benefits or reduce some of the negative side effects.

In integrated treatment, therefore, the psychiatrist usually tries to start with one type of treatment, see how it works, and then add another treatment if necessary. In integrated treatment, one could start with either medication or psychotherapy and then add the other, or start with both medication and psychotherapy at the same time. However, sequencing is a complex issue (Beitman et al. 2003).

Diagnosis matters, because with patients who have depression or anxiety, providing medication first and dampening down symptoms might allow the patient to more fully participate in a form of psychotherapy. Similarly, with patients with a psychotic disorder, the patient may be suspicious, hallucinating, delusional, or manic and would need to be medicated first to feel more comfortable sitting and talking with a physician.

A good clinician will fully appreciate that things are not black and white. A suspicious, paranoid patient is not going to take medication prescribed by a clinician unless there is a good doctor–patient alliance. The patient needs to feel at least a little bit hopeful that the doctor means well and that the medicine is going to make the patient feel better—and not poison him or her. This alliance is based on talk between the patient and doctor. This talk could be viewed is part of supportive psychotherapy, interpersonal psychotherapy, or a type of cognitive-behavioral psychotherapy. So, one could argue that medication and psychotherapy are not really being sequenced but that they are integral.

With that said, in determining a treatment plan the psychiatry resident should discuss with the patient all proven, effective types of treatment. Such types of treatment should at least be discussed, even if the clinician cannot provide the treatment himself or herself. The patient should nevertheless be informed of the options that are available.

The patient should be provided with the information about the kinds of psychotropic medication and psychotherapy the clinician is considering: whether one or the other or both should be used, whether one should start before the other, and if not why not. Patients arrive with expectations about what the psychiatrist will do: some are afraid of doctors being "pill pushers"; some have had good experiences with medications and want the doctor to give them pills to help take away painful symptoms; some view doctors as uncaring people who are too busy to really listen to patients and just want to write a prescription or order a consultation to send the patient off; and some view doctors as money-seeking practitioners who are just in it to get rich. Although many of these are negative constructs, most patients are very respectful and hopeful that the psychiatrist can help. After all, that is probably why they come to the psychiatrist's office, tell their stories, and hope that the clinician can figure out the problem. Addressing these constructs could certainly facilitate the treatment process.

Starting With Medication

The diagnosis is critical to the resident's decision whether or not to medicate in the beginning of treatment. It is important to determine how the patient feels about medication. If he or she is frightened, does not have the money to pay for medication, or has concomitant medical conditions for which more information is needed from the primary care physician, then holding off on prescribing early would be advisable. On the other hand, if the patient has a diagnosis amenable to medication (e.g., recurrent major depression) and has not been taking antidepressant medication since the last episode, it might be very reasonable to consider prescribing antidepressant medication in the very early stages of the treatment plan. One might consider providing antidepressant medication and discussing possible side effects, what to expect by taking the medication, and what might be added later (another augmenting agent or psychotherapy). In addition, there may be somatic problems that need to be treated sooner if the antidepressant does not address some problems such as falling asleep, staying asleep, or daytime anxiety.

If the patient then continues with the antidepressant medication and starts feeling less sad and hopeless, he or she may begin to tell the clinician about stressors or triggers at the start of the depressive episode. If there are issues that relate to family members, the psychotherapy might be most suitably administered as couples therapy; or with problems in organization or work relationships, cognitive-behavioral treatment might be most suitable. Psychiatrists often like to see the patient have fewer somatic problems and fewer acute problems before moving away from focusing on medication and concentrating more on problem solving.

Setting certainly plays an important part in sequencing. For example, if the first contact is in the emergency setting, medication might be provided first before psychotherapy just because the symptoms presented are usually more acute and the follow-up care will be provided by another physician. Similarly, in the inpatient setting, where stays are quite short, medication might be provided before a course of psychotherapy.

But in the outpatient setting, where the resident will be providing integrated treatment, the diagnosis, the patient's expectations, and the acuity of symptoms are probably the largest factors in determining whether medication will be provided at the outset.

Even though medication might be warranted, another issue for the resident to consider is whether it might be more judicious to wait and see. What this means is that the patient might look different or present differently after a few sessions. What seems like anxiety early on might settle down very quickly as the patient gets to know the resident, and other symptoms or problems might emerge that might be more amenable to other types of treatment. What seems like an adjustment disorder with depressed mood may turn out to be an adjustment disorder that may clear after several psychotherapy sessions, or it may turn out to be major depression, for which medication is warranted.

Sometimes the clinician is unsure of the working diagnosis, and in such cases it might be prudent to wait before prescribing medication. Once medication has been started, it is harder to pull back or stop it. If a patient develops an untoward side effect, it might be more difficult to persuade the patient to try a higher dosage of the medication or even a different class of drug.

Starting With Psychotherapy

If a form of psychotherapy is indicated, it is usually helpful to begin with education about the patient's diagnosis, what kinds of treatment are indicated, and if psychotherapy is recommended, what type. Patients like to know how long the treatment will last, what they should expect, whether they will be somehow different after it is complete, and what happens if the treatment is not successful. Patients may come in with an experience of themselves or family members after a form of psychotherapy. It is helpful for the clinician to know about that and to put the currently recommended form of therapy in context with what the patient may have already experienced or have some knowledge about.

What is very difficult for psychiatry residents is that although they need to educate and inform patients, they themselves probably do not have the clinical experience or background to fully answer all the questions posed. Furthermore, the resident might not have actually completed a form of psychotherapy with a patient with a similar problem and so may be anxious himself about whether or not he can even deliver the proper type of care. Often a supervisor is helping the resident through the first couple of cases of a type of psychotherapy, and even though the patient might be aware of this level of supervision, the resident might be in the unenviable position of feeling very alone in the provision of care.

It is therefore to be expected if the resident does not feel confident that a form of psychotherapy is definitely going to work or be successful. It is a difficult position to be in for the resident and for the patient, but just recognizing that this is the situation may help the resident request more supervision and may allow the patient to work more closely in partnership with the resident. Patients who choose teaching hospitals usually realize that the opportunity to work with bright, energetic trainees is a plus, even if they are not as seasoned and experienced as others in practice. The financial benefit of seeing a trainee might be a determining factor, or the availability and proximity to the institution may be the limiting issues.

Residents should not feel that they have to be able to deliver the most perfect form of psychotherapy. What they need to do is do the best they can for their patient and realize that it is a training and teaching situation.

There are, of course, situations for the provision of psychotherapy and medication in which consultation or referral is warranted because the patient is not doing well, the resident realizes that he or she cannot provide the needed care, or a combination of both. These decisions should be discussed with the supervisor, and the emphasis should always be in favor of providing what is best for the patient. Weighing these issues and making sure that the resident is not referring based on his or her own novice anxiety is very complex and is part of the training process.

When psychotherapy is begun initially, the focus is usually on dynamic issues and principles. In addition, CBT is a very important type of treatment for a wide range of disorders, including anxiety, depression, and substance abuse. When a patient's symptoms begin to emerge that might be treated with medication, it is up to the resident to determine the risks and benefits of treating those symptoms with medication versus allowing the dynamic process to evolve. Again, the diagnosis is critical. The working diagnosis should constantly be revisited. What started out as mild depression could over time develop into moderate or severe major depression that needs to be treated with medication. Continuing a form of psychotherapy without at least raising the possibility of using antidepressants might be quite risky. Similarly, a patient with a history of posttraumatic stress disorder might be presenting with mild symptoms of mood problems, and with psychotherapy there could be a reviewing of the initial trauma that could result in disequilibrium in anxiety and mood symptoms. Reassessment might lead to the conclusion that there needs to be an addition of medication to the psychotherapy regimen.

> **Competency:** The psychiatry resident must be able to demonstrate the ability to form a working therapeutic alliance at the beginning of treatment.

> **Competency:** The psychiatry resident must be able to demonstrate the ability to appreciate the issues that involve sequencing of medication (and/or other medical treatments) and psychotherapy.

Maintenance

It is difficult for most people to maintain anything—optimum weight, good grades, high job performance, etc. We all have to work at maintenance: our dentists need to send us reminders about getting regular checkups; our cars have lights in the dashboard that come on to tell us that service needs to be performed; and so on. Most of us get bored or tired of doing the same thing day in and day out. We get complacent about how things are going; we want to see what will happen if we stop doing something that we regularly do; we want to see if there are cheaper or easier ways to get the same result.

A critical phase of treatment begins when the patient has become stable on medication and psychotherapy. The resident might be quite pleased about how the patient is doing, and so might the patient. But taking pills every day, coming to see the resident regularly, and paying the pharmacy and the clinic when one is feeling relatively well might become triggers for the patient to want to make changes. It is therefore an important time for the resident, who might be very pleased with what she has accomplished with the patient, to realize that she has to work very hard to make sure the patient's good health continues.

During the maintenance phase, for example, it is a good time to ask about sexual side effects. In the early phases of taking medication when the patient might have been quite depressed and anxious, low libido or decreased interest in sex might not have been so important to the patient. As the patient begins to feel well and his significant other sees that he is doing better with life activities, sex might again become important. If the medication prescribed by the resident has the potential to alter the patient's sex drive, it is important to raise that as an issue. The patient might not want to bring this issue up to the resident because he might realize that the resident is going to urge the patient to keep taking the medication. The patient might therefore start cutting down on the dosage to see what will happen.

Another issue during the maintenance phase is paying for medication and treatment. Most patients at least have to make a copayment for these forms of treatment. It might become a burden for patients to be paying for these forms of treatment, so they might be thinking about what can be cut from the regimen. Again, it is better for the resident to be proactive about bringing up these issues and to work in partnership with the patient on these matters.

Family problems that are sometimes put on the back burner during a patient's acute presentation of symptoms move more to the epicenter during maintenance treatment. Marital problems, parent–child issues, or financial troubles may all resurface as the patient starts improving. Bringing other family members into sessions with the patient might be helpful. If the patient is receiving integrated treatment—medication and psychotherapy—the clinician and the patient can determine when and how these collateral partners might be brought into the care.

Adherence

It is very difficult for anyone to strictly adhere to a treatment plan, especially taking medication. Most people do not like to take medication. How many people actually take a full course of antibiotics? Often, as they begin to feel better, they stop taking the medication. The track record in primary care with antidepressants is bleak—after 6 months, most patients are not taking the full dosage of antidepressant medication that was initially prescribed by the primary care doctor.

Nonadherence with medication regimens can take many forms: not getting prescriptions filled; not taking medications as prescribed, either taking too many pills or too few, or not taking them on the right schedule; taking medication while also using alcohol or other drugs; stopping medication before the agreed-on time. With regard to psychotherapeutic treatment, nonadherence might mean not keeping appointments, canceling appointments at the last minute, arriving late, not paying for treatment, not bringing family members or other participants to treatment, not completing homework assignments, etc.

There are also other factors related to the patient's psychopathology that may affect nonadherence: paranoia, suspiciousness, or psychosis; substance abuse; cognitive deficits, such as poor memory; or severe depression that prompts psychomotor agitation and feelings of hopelessness or worthlessness.

What can the psychiatry resident do to improve adherence with the prescribed treatment of medication and psychotherapy? Some suggestions are listed below.

- Most patients appreciate education about the form of treatment they are receiving. Although written materials are helpful, for certain types of patients it might be more useful to use the telephone to provide information. Fact sheets about the medication and psychotherapy are good adjuncts. Web sites, handouts, books, and pamphlets are often useful. Although it is true that some patients will be frightened by what they read and might feel that they are getting all the possible side effects that are listed, it is probably more important that they receive the information, and they can then can discuss it with the resident.

- Some patients will benefit from joining support groups or local chapters of organizations for those with the same or similar disorder. Therefore it might be useful to refer patients to the National Alliance for the Mentally Ill (NAMI), the Depression and Bipolar Support Alliance (DBSA), Alcoholics Anonymous (AA), Narcotics Anonymous (NA), or Al-Anon.

- Bringing family members into certain sessions might be very useful. Asking the patient's partner—spouse, girlfriend, or boyfriend—about how best to help the patient adhere to treatment can be beneficial.

- It is important to continue to ask patients about side effects and the state of their general medical health. Patients will realize that the clinician is continually vigilant about their medications and wants to make sure that things are going well. When might be a good time to decrease the dosage or stop the medication is a good topic for conversation. Sometimes patients might think that the clinician wants them to take the medication indefinitely, when that might not be the case at all.

- The pharmaceutical companies are doing a lot of direct-to-consumer advertising. If there is a big media blitz about a specific medication, it might be useful to ask patients what they have heard and what they are thinking. It might be a good time to talk about why the new medication on the market might or might not be good for the patient.
- Many patients might want to take alternative or complementary medications or substances obtained from health food stores or over the Internet. There are various reasons why more and more people are looking to use such substances, but it is important to ask about such issues on a regular basis. A substance that a patient is using as a supplement might not have an adverse impact on the main form of psychiatric treatment, but it could have an effect, and so it is important to know about.
- To treat a concomitant medical problem, the patient's primary care physician or specialty physician might have prescribed a new medication that is interacting with the psychotropic medication. It is important to know this so that the dosage of the psychotropic medication (or the medication itself) can be changed before the patient stops taking it altogether, which could lead to an escalation in psychiatric symptoms.
- Packaging interventions—such as using daily or weekly dosing, liquid or sublingual preparations, blister packs, etc.—might be useful for some patients as a behavioral strategy.
- First impressions of the resident are important. If the resident seems competent and confident, the patient usually feels better about adhering to treatment.
- When patients drop out of psychodynamic treatment, reasons often include a weaker therapeutic alliance, less of a focus on the patient's affect, and less supportive and dynamic work during the sessions (Piper et al. 1999).

> **Competency:** The psychiatry resident must be able to demonstrate knowledge of the factors that are important for the individual patient to maintain and adhere to a treatment regimen.

Conclusion

It is very difficult to know, based on the literature, how best to sequence medication and psychotherapy for patients in general. Providing a good working diagnosis, developing a treatment plan that is agreed to by both the patient and the resident, and continuing to evaluate how the patient is doing are all ways to improve the course of care. Although beginning the treatment is hard, it is also difficult to manage the maintenance phase of integrated treatment, as well as helping the patient to adhere to ongoing, regular use of medication and psychotherapy. It is important for psychiatry residents to ask patients how they are doing, even when they appear to be doing well, because that is the time when patients might try changes in treatment on their own, without partnering with the resident about such changes. Listening for and attending to these difficult periods in treatment are crucial when the resident is trying to administer optimal integrated care.

There are high-risk times for nonadherence to treatment: for example, at the beginning of treatment before the doctor–patient relationship has been solidified and before the onset of a good therapeutic alliance. In addition, it often takes some time before a medication or psychotherapy begins to take effect or for the patient or family to see results. For those who are impatient or who are looking for reasons not to continue in treatment, this could be viewed as a high-risk time. Later on, there may be fears of dependence or drug addiction, and transference issues between the patient and physician may be reasons for adherence problems.

Psychotherapy and pharmacotherapy can be adjuncts to one another. While the medication is being started and the dosage adjusted, it is helpful for the clinician to help the patient stay engaged in pleasurable activities and functions that had been important parts of the patient's life. Medication clinics are very useful for many patients as a way to decrease stigma and provide education and as a way to give support. Personalized attention from clinicians, nurses, and other mental health providers, either by telephone or e-mail, also appears to be very effective.

The resident should assume that adherence to psychotherapy and pharmacotherapy will be difficult for most patients. The patient's adherence to medical and mental health treatment should be reviewed. At each session, a significant amount of time should be spent on monitoring symptoms and checking on issues related to adherence, especially in the early stages of treatment. Problems that the patient is having with obtaining the medication, taking the medication, getting to appointments, doing homework assignments, and arranging for support from friends and family members should all be explored (Wetherell 2003). Any problems with these issues should be identified proactively, and problem solving should be part of the treatment. More frequent contact—either by telephone, by office visits, or by e-mail—should be explored. Bringing in family members or other support persons should be investigated. If the patient has cognitive deficits, having family members or others help would be an important factor for success.

It is imperative that the resident help to solve problems and find out about the issues without appearing threatening or angry about the non-adherence. The goal of treatment is for the patient to be able to self-monitor and provide ways to improve adherence on his or her own, for both medication and psychotherapy. It is important for the patient to feel that any problems can be addressed and discussed with the resident to make the treatment as successful as possible.

References

Beitman BD, Blinder BJ, Thase ME, et al: Integrating Psychotherapy and Pharmacotherapy: Dissolving the Mind-Brain Barrier. New York, WW Norton, 2003

Burnand Y, Andreoli A, Kolatte E, et al: Psychodynamic psychotherapy and clomipramine in the treatment of major depression. Psychiatr Serv 53:585–590, 2002

de Jonghe F, Kool S, van Aalst G, et al: Combining psychotherapy and antidepressants in the treatment of depression. J Affect Disord 64:217–229, 2001

Dunner DL: Acute and maintenance treatment for chronic depression. J Clin Psychiatry 62 (suppl 6):10–16, 2001

Hirschfeld RM, Dunner DL, Keitner G, et al: Does psychosocial functioning improve independent of depressive symptoms? A comparison of nefazodone, psychotherapy, and their combination. Biol Psychiatry 51:123–133, 2002

Keller MB, McCullough JP, Klein DN, et al: A comparison of nefazodone, the cognitive behavioral-analysis system of psychotherapy, and their combination for the treatment of chronic depression. N Engl J Med 342:1462–1470, 2000

Piper WE, Ogrodniczuk JS, Joyce AS, et al: Prediction of dropping out in time-limited, interpretive individual psychotherapy. Psychotherapy 36:114–122, 1999

Roose SP: Psychodynamic therapy and medication: can treatments in conflict be integrated? in Integrated Treatment of Psychiatric Disorders. Edited by Kay J (Review of Psychiatry series; Oldham JM and Riba MB, series eds). Washington, DC, American Psychiatric Publishing, 2001, pp 31–49

Wetherell JL, Unutzer J: Adherence to treatment for geriatric depression and anxiety. CNS Spectr 8 (12 suppl 3):48–59, 2003

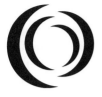

5

Termination in Integrated Treatment

Integrated treatment may continue indefinitely in some cases of serious or recurrent major mental disorder. However, in most cases, the treatment will be terminated at some point. Termination in integrated treatment could mean either simultaneous termination of pharmacotherapy and psychotherapy (although this is rarely done) or sequenced termination, with either pharmacotherapy or psychotherapy being terminated first and the other modality terminated later.

The simultaneous termination of both modalities is frequently forced by the patient, either by requesting it and discussing it with the treating psychiatrist, or just by not showing up for treatment. As Bender and Messner (2003) point out, these patients are not terminating but are quitting treatment. Patients may either feel that they have improved sufficiently or that the returns of therapy have been significantly diminishing (Makover 2004). Another rather unfortunate possible reason for termination of treatment is the patient's lack of resources to continue in treatment: either the third-party payer decides that the cost outweighs the benefit (Makover 2004) or covers only a predetermined number of sessions per specific disorder or condition; or the patient, paying out of pocket for treatment, runs out of money. A special case of termination occurs during residency training: many patients treated by residents are transferred to another resident after the treating resident leaves the program. Although this is not a true *treatment* termination, it is a termination of a therapeutic relationship, and as such it also needs to be carefully planned and executed. Finally, one should realize that the decision to refer the patient for therapy after an initial period of pharmacotherapy (medication management) while pharmacotherapy continues (split arrangement) may be viewed by the patient as termination and should be handled in a similar fashion in some cases.

Termination of any treatment should always be planned well ahead, preferably several months in advance. Makover (2004) even suggests that it begins at the beginning of treatment (or at least its planning probably should). The sequencing of termination is a complicated process that depends on various factors, including the diagnosis; severity of illness; efficacy and outcome of integrated treatment so far; the psychotherapeutic modality used; overall treatment goals; treatment goals of each modality; the patient's preferences, beliefs, and misconceptions; medication side effects; and, unfortunately, financial resources.

An example of the complexity of termination sequencing in integrated treatment is provided by the case of major depression. In a single episode of major depression, one may consider terminating the course of cognitive-behavioral therapy after 12 sessions and significant improvement, but continuing antidepressant treatment for another several months to achieve the recommended 6- to 9-month period of stable improvement. In another case of a single episode of major depression, one may consider terminating antidepressant treatment after 9 months of stable improvement while continuing supportive psychotherapy addressing adjustment to a new job or marital problems. In the case of recurrent major depression, one may terminate psychotherapy and continue antidepressant treatment indefinitely.

Thoughtful use of either pharmacotherapy or psychotherapy could be helpful when terminating the other kind of therapy. Psychotherapy could be extremely helpful at the time of terminating pharmacotherapy. It could help dissolve some of the patient's anxieties about stopping medication and being on his own. It could also help with the occasional recurrence of some symptoms (however, one should not confuse the occasional transitional symptoms such as anxiety with a true relapse or recurrence of the illness).

One should be aware that termination of either pharmacotherapy or psychotherapy is frequently difficult and may trigger strong transference and countertransference. Termination of pharmacotherapy, psychotherapy, or both preferably occurs after a mutual agreement and in collaboration with the patient. However, at times a resident may be forced to terminate one or both treatment modalities unilaterally (e.g., for lack of adherence to treatment, continuous substance abuse, or failure to pay for treatment or after determining that the patient may be a "therapeutic lifer"). Gabbard (2004) points out that "in most states, it is perfectly legal to discontinue treatment provided that suicidality or danger to others has been carefully assessed." One should provide the notice of termination in writing and list potential treaters in case the patient would like to seek treatment in the future (Gabbard 2004). It may be useful to emphasize the necessity of continuing pharmacotherapy in cases of highly recurrent or chronic disorders.

The decision about sequencing the termination of pharmacotherapy and psychotherapy in integrated treatment is *relatively* easier than in collaborative or split treatment, because it involves only two parties.

> **Competency:** The psychiatry resident should be able to demonstrate the factors that are helpful in terminating care with patients.

Terminating Pharmacotherapy First

The discussion about terminating pharmacotherapy quite frequently starts at the beginning of pharmacotherapy. This discussion is frequently triggered by the patient's uneasiness over taking psychotropic medication. Besides asking about the side effects, one of the first questions many patients ask is, "How long will I have to take this medication?" An honest answer, including the possibility that the psychiatrist does not know or is not sure, should follow. The initial discussion of treatment and formulation of the treatment plan should always include the goals of each treatment modality and the possible best time for termination of each treatment type (Beitman et al. 2003). This discussion should be specific (as much as possible) and clear. For instance, specifying the duration of pharmacotherapy in case of the first episode of major depression is relatively easy. The patient should know that she will continue taking the antidepressant (at its full dosage) for 6–9 months after reaching remission, which in lay terms means after starting to feel and function well. The issue of counting the duration of the continuation of pharmacotherapy from the time of feeling well is important. It can frequently take 2–3 months to reach full remission. Patients may start to press for termination of medication in another 3 months—clearly an insufficient time.

The suggested length of pharmacotherapy varies from disorder to disorder and depends on various factors (chronicity, severity, and recurrence of the disorder; previous response and adherence to medication; family history; presence of stresses; and others). In many cases the discontinuation of medication is not a simple process accomplished by simply saying, "No more pills starting tomorrow." Many psychotropic medications need to be discontinued gradually; some, over a period of a few days; and some, over a period of a few weeks (e.g., high dosages of alprazolam). Because polypharmacy has become quite common, discontinuation of medications could become quite a complicated task. Take an example of a patient treated with an antidepressant, a mood stabilizer, and a hypnotic. Which one should be stopped first? Second? We suggest that one never discontinue more than one medication at the same time. The sequencing of the discontinuation of several medications should be individualized, and all the general suggestions about discontinuation could be applied to each particular medication.

The initial planning of pharmacotherapy termination should also include the discussion of what is going to happen with psychotherapy—how to stagger the discontinuation of both modalities. The patient should clearly understand that terminating pharmacotherapy *does not* inevitably mean terminating psychotherapy (the resident should not forget that we are discussing the termination of pharmacotherapy while psychotherapy continues). Finally, the initial discussion may include the issues of recurrence of symptoms and follow-up after pharmacotherapy termination. However, these issues may come up more frequently during the process of termination itself.

Beitman et al. (2003) and others suggest announcing termination early, at least 3–6 months ahead. Mischoulon and colleagues (2000) also suggest the general timeline of 3–6 months for announcing the termination. They also provide several suggestions for ameliorating the change of psychopharmacologist, which may be adapted for termination of pharmacotherapy.

These modified suggestions include informing the patient that symptoms may worsen transiently after the termination, reminding the patient of termination during each visit in the termination phase and allowing the patient to verbalize his or her feelings, and even using a standardized protocol for transfer and termination (Mischoulon et al. 2000).

We believe that the discussion of medication termination should also include further clinical issues such as the following:

1. The possibility of physiological as well as psychological withdrawal symptoms (not only with benzodiazepines, but also with some selective serotonin reuptake inhibitors and other psychotropic medications) after stopping the medication. The discussion should include the timeline of these symptoms (e.g., withdrawal symptoms after the discontinuation of some benzodiazepines with long half-lives may be

delayed for 1–2 weeks, whereas withdrawal symptoms associated with alprazolam may occur almost immediately) and a plan for their management.

2. The chance of increased suicidality during the discontinuation phase of some medications (see the recent U.S. Food and Drug Administration warning about the discontinuation of antidepressants) or after the discontinuation of lithium (e.g., Tondo et al. 1997).

3. Aftercare monitoring of withdrawal symptoms, recurrence symptoms, suicidality, and other clinical issues (which, in the case of continuing psychotherapy should not be difficult). In case any unusual symptoms occur, patients should be encouraged to contact the resident as soon as possible and at any time. Some residents may prefer being contacted via e-mail (for guidelines see Silk and Yager 2003).

4. Avoidance of triggers of various symptoms. This means maintaining a healthy lifestyle, including avoiding or limiting the use of alcohol, caffeine, and tobacco; exercising; and getting regular and sufficient sleep.

5. Reassuring the patient that the issues of medication discontinuation could be freely discussed during several subsequent psychotherapy sessions. However, the issue of medication discontinuation should not become a dominating concern in continuing psychotherapy.

Residents should always discuss the termination plan with their clinical and psychotherapy supervisors.

> **Competency:** The psychiatry resident should be able to demonstrate the skills and knowledge to terminate with patients regarding pharmacotherapy when both pharmacotherapy and psychotherapy were provided by the resident.

Terminating Psychotherapy First

Termination of psychotherapy in integrated treatment, while pharmacotherapy continues, is usually a more complicated task than terminating pharmacotherapy first. Psychotherapy may be terminated, as mutually agreed, after certain goals of psychotherapy have been achieved (probably more frequently in a course of cognitive-behavioral therapy, brief psychotherapy, or supportive psychotherapy than in long-term psychodynamic psychotherapy). Termination of psychotherapy in integrated treatment may also be forced by various circumstances, such as 1) the patient or therapist feeling that there is no value in continuing psychotherapy; 2) relocation of either the patient or the physician, including graduation or change of rotation of the resident (however, this also forces simultaneous termination of pharmacotherapy); or 3) economic reasons (either the third-party payer refuses to pay for more sessions or the patient paying out of pocket runs out of money, or the number of sessions was predetermined from the beginning).

Similar to the termination of pharmacotherapy, initial discussion of treatment and formulation of the treatment plan should always include the goals of psychotherapy and the best possible time for termination (Beitman et al. 2003). The time frame of psychotherapy termination should always be individualized. The fact that the timing of termination may be predetermined (a number of sessions agreed on from the beginning or forced by the third-party payer) does not necessarily make the termination easier and does not mean that it should not be carefully planned and executed. Termination should be discussed for several sessions before the last psychotherapy session. Ideally, one would allow something similar to the 3–6 months in the case of pharmacotherapy. However, some psychotherapy modalities (cognitive-behavioral therapy and brief psychotherapy) have shorter durations and thus do not allow for such a long termination process. It is generally recommended that the patient should be informed about the planned date of termination at the beginning of psychotherapy in cases of forced termination with a known termination date (e.g., the resident knows that she will be leaving the service or training program in a year).

The patient's readiness for termination should be regularly assessed during the termination phase of psychotherapy. The termination process frequently brings up a number of transference issues. Some patients may "start flooding each remaining session with a barrage of new material and push themselves to discuss previously avoided material" (Bender and Messner 2003, p. 297). The patient may become openly hostile or angry, may miss sessions or come late, and may regress or even decompensate (Bender and Messner 2003). Many training programs witness an increase of regressing or decompensated patients, who continue taking medications, during the May–June period when residents terminate their long-term cases before departing from residency. A special issue in integrated treatment may be the threat of noncompliance or lack of adherence with pharmacotherapy regimens. It is well known that psychotherapy induces stronger compliance with pharmacotherapy and with the combination of treatment modalities (e.g., in depression; see Pampallona et al. 2004). When psychotherapy is being terminated for whatever reason and the treatment plan calls for continuing medication for various reasons (mainly the prevention of relapse or attenuation of residual symptoms), the patient may threaten to skip or stop taking the medication. The dangers of terminating medication—especially terminating it suddenly— need to be included in the discussion of termination. However, the continuation of pharmacotherapy (the reader should not forget that we are discussing terminating psychotherapy while pharmacotherapy is continuing) could provide some help in terminating psychotherapy. The doctor– patient relationship is not completely terminated. Also, pharmacotherapy sessions may be used for some therapeutic support, for prevention of decompensation, or for addressing the decompensation after the termination of psychotherapy.

The process of termination may also trigger (or be triggered by) various countertransference issues. These issues may interfere with a careful assessment of the patient's readiness to terminate psychotherapy. Gabbard (2004) points out several countertransference issues that could play a role in planning and executing psychotherapy termination by any therapist, including residents. Residents may overestimate or idealize psychotherapy and avoid conducting a proper, well-planned termination. Residents may also hold on to patients for their own needs. Certain patients may even enhance the therapist's self-esteem, making the termination difficult if not impossible. However, the countertransference may also force premature termination, because some patients may arouse contempt, boredom, hatred, and anger in residents (Gabbard 2004). The resident should always discuss the termination issues in supervision.

Termination of psychotherapy may also lead to an increase in the permeability of boundaries (Gabbard 2004). Patients may be inclined to ask more personal questions and might offer gifts or hugs. However, such issues might not arise as frequently when terminating psychotherapy in integrated treatment while pharmacotherapy continues. Nevertheless, residents should be aware of the possibility of these boundary issues. Should the gift be accepted as a well-meant symbol of termination, or should it be rejected and discussed? Should the hug be accepted or rejected? These are complicated issues that need to be addressed on an individual basis and in a frame of proper supervision.

We recommend that the termination of psychotherapy be well planned in advance and structured according to the following guidelines:

1. Termination of psychotherapy is announced and planned either from the very beginning in the case of time-limited therapies, or several months in advance in the case of long-term psychotherapy.
2. The patient's feelings, worries, and transference about and reaction to psychotherapy termination are regularly explored, discussed, and

addressed. The patient should be actively invited to verbalize his or her feelings about termination during several termination sessions.

3. In some cases the patient could be offered several intermittent, as-needed termination sessions between pharmacotherapy appointments. Psychotherapy may be tapered off this way (e.g., from once a week to once a month to occasionally to none) while pharmacotherapy continues.

4. Possible decompensation, acting out, recurrence of symptoms, and occurrence of suicidality should be carefully monitored.

5. Medication adjustment or addition may occasionally be offered to manage various symptoms or decompensation during the termination.

6. Increased attention to adherence to the originally prescribed medication regimen (i.e., continuing pharmacotherapy) is recommended.

7. The patient should be reassured that the doctor–patient relationship is not terminated and that she could bring up some therapeutic issues during the course of continuing pharmacotherapy. However, one should be careful that this does not sabotage the entire process of termination and that the patient does not surreptitiously bring the therapy back. Junior residents have a tendency to continue psychotherapy during the medication review appointments.

8. Just as during termination of pharmacotherapy, patients should be educated that avoiding stressors such as emotional conflicts could be helpful during termination of psychotherapy.

9. The resident should be aware of the increased possibility of boundary violations during termination of psychotherapy.

10. The resident should always seek proper and frequent supervision to address all termination issues.

> **Competency:** The psychiatry resident should be able to demonstrate the skills and knowledge to terminate with patients regarding psychotherapy when both pharmacotherapy and psychotherapy were provided by the resident.

A final word about termination: Contrary to previously held views, termination does not necessarily mean permanent ending. Bender and Messner (2003) point out that "while it is important to view a therapy's termination as a completion of a piece of work, this does not mean that future (professional) meetings cannot occur" (p. 306). Many psychiatrists and therapist explicitly invite their patients to call them in the future—for example, in cases of setbacks or relapse.

Terminating Pharmacotherapy and Psychotherapy at the Same Time

Simultaneous termination of pharmacotherapy and psychotherapy in integrated treatment in everyday practice is usually rare. However, simultaneous termination of both pharmacotherapy and psychotherapy occurs fairly frequently in residency training programs—at the time when residents terminate their cases before graduating or changing services. Usually, this is not a true termination of treatment or treatment modality as discussed in this chapter so far, but a termination of a doctor–patient relationship and transfer to another resident. This process could be quite demanding, taxing, and difficult.

Simultaneous termination stirs up similar feelings as termination of psychotherapy or pharmacotherapy. Patients may feel angry, devastated, and abandoned. For some patients, this is the déjà vu experience they go through several times while being treated in training programs.

Transfer to another resident should be carefully planned, and the planning should start several (3–6) months in advance. The plan should include all issues about termination of psychotherapy discussed in this chapter. In addition, it may be helpful to arrange an early meeting with the new resident (Mischoulon et al. 2000). The departing resident may emphasize the benefits of the new physician, such as a fresh outlook, new ideas, etc. (Mischoulon et al. 2000). The departing resident may also offer a few scheduled telephone sessions during this period of transition (Bender and Messner 2003) and offer to be available over the telephone or by e-mail in case of crises. However, the boundaries and rules of these contacts must be set at the beginning. We have also found the use of support staff helpful in this process of transition. A good, empathic support staff could provide a symbol of some permanence contrasting with the yearly changing residents and may thus help to smooth the transition.

The transfer rules apply not only to transfers within the residency training program but also to any mutually agreeable and planned transfer of the patient in clinical practice. The departing (due to retirement, relocation, illness, or other reasons) psychiatrist should provide the patient with a referral and then should apply rules similar to those discussed for transfer within the residency training program. These recommendations similarly apply to termination due to patient relocation.

The (infrequent) simultaneous termination of pharmacotherapy and psychotherapy would require combining the recommendations about the termination of both pharmacotherapy and psychotherapy. However, we do not recommend an actual simultaneous termination, because of a number of possible complications and difficulties associated with this process. Instead we recommend sequencing the termination of integrated treatment, starting with either pharmacotherapy or psychotherapy. As pointed out, the sequencing should be individualized and depends on numerous clinical, personal, and economic factors.

Transfer to another therapist or true simultaneous termination also requires addressing the posttermination psychiatrist–patient boundary issues (Malmquist and Notman 2001). The posttermination time is a period of increased probability and propensity for boundary violations, which can range from accepting improper gifts to emotional or sexual involvement. The discussion of proper posttreatment boundaries (basically the same as boundaries that exist during treatment) should be always included in termination planning.

> **Competency:** The psychiatry resident should be able to demonstrate the skills and knowledge to terminate with patients regarding both pharmacotherapy and psychotherapy when both pharmacotherapy and psychotherapy were provided by the resident.

Termination is an important part of any therapeutic process. Its proper planning and execution should always be a part of proper, competent treatment.

References

Beitman BD, Blinder BJ, Thase ME, et al: Integrating Psychotherapy and Pharmacotherapy: Dissolving the Mind-Brain Barrier. New York, WW Norton 2003

Bender S, Messner E: Becoming a Therapist: What Do I Say, and Why? New York, Guilford, 2003

Gabbard GO: Long-Term Psychodynamic Psychotherapy: A Basic Text (Core Competency in Psychotherapy Series). Arlington, VA, American Psychiatric Publishing, 2004

Makover RB: Treatment Planning for Psychotherapists: A Practical Guide to Better Outcomes, 2nd Edition. Arlington, VA, American Psychiatric Publishing, 2004

Malmquist CP, Notman MT: Psychiatrist-patient boundary issues following treatment termination. Am J Psychiatry 158:1010–1018, 2001

Mischoulon D, Rosenbaum JF, Messner E: Transfer to a new psychopharmacologist: its effect on patients. Academic Psychiatry 24:156–163, 2000

Pampallona S, Bollini P, Tibaldi G, et al: Combined pharmacotherapy and psychological treatment for depression: a systematic review. Arch Gen Psychiatry 61:714–719, 2004

Silk KR, Yager J: Suggested guidelines for e-mail communication in psychiatric practice. J Clin Psychiatry 64:799–806, 2003

Tondo L, Jamison KR, Baldessarini RJ: Effect of lithium maintenance on suicidal behavior in major mood disorders. Ann N Y Acad Sci 836:339–351, 1997

Part II

Split Treatment

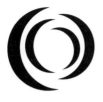

Selection of Medication, Psychotherapy, and Clinicians in Split Treatment

There are several different ways that a resident can find himself or herself providing split treatment for a patient. Some of the possible circumstances include the following:

A. The patient is seen by the resident for a psychiatric evaluation. In the course of the evaluation, the resident determines that it would be best for the patient to see another clinician (usually a social worker or psychologist) for psychotherapy, and the resident would see the patient for medication and medical issues related to the treatment.
B. The patient is seen by the resident for a psychiatric evaluation. In the course of the evaluation, the patient tells the resident that she is already seeing a therapist and was referred for medication. The resident, if he feels that medication is warranted, would be the provider of the psychotropic medication and other pertinent medical issues.
C. The patient is already being seen by a therapist. A primary care physician or other physician has been treating the patient with psychotropic medication, but the patient is not improving, so the physician

sends the patient to the clinic/resident for more expert evaluation and treatment.

D. The patient is seeing a resident for integrated treatment—psychotherapy and medication—but the psychotherapy part of the care will end (both the patient and resident agree that psychotherapy is no longer needed; insurance benefits changed; the patient can no longer afford to see both a therapist and the resident; the patient decides that she does not want psychotherapy, etc.), so the resident continues to see the patient for medication and medical management.

In all the situations outlined above, there are particular decisions that the resident and supervisor must make in determining the proper care for the patient: what the resident is able and competent to provide; the timing of the combination and sequencing of medication and psychotherapy; and who the resident should refer the patient to based on the need for a certain type of psychotherapy.

The issues and tasks noted above are some of the most difficult for even seasoned clinicians. The resident must often make these assessments in a single evaluation while also trying to formulate a diagnosis and a treatment plan, assess strengths and weaknesses of the treatment plan and obstacles to its implementation, and ascertain access to care.

In this chapter, we highlight some of the specific issues that the resident needs to consider in the various scenarios described above, realizing that these situations are very fluid and can easily shift based on a wide variety of factors. This process is very complex and difficult, particularly because it is triangulated: it involves the patient, the resident, and another clinician who will be providing the primary treatment.

Scenario A

In this circumstance, the resident makes a decision, based on the evaluation, to refer the patient to another clinician for psychotherapy while continuing to see the patient for medication. What are the factors that would lead the resident to this recommendation?

The patient's history is quite important. The patient might tell the resident that she has had this type of split treatment in the past and has done well with it. The resident might want to ask the patient why she did not go back to the former treaters. It could be that the patient moved, the previous treaters are no longer available, it is inconvenient for the patient to seek treatment with the previous providers, or the patient has a different type of insurance plan. It is important to discover these factors to clarify the reasons why the patient is seeking new clinicians.

The resident might feel that the patient would benefit from being seen frequently, but the resident's schedule does not allow such frequency. For example, the patient may have a diagnosis of major depression and mild, recurrent, and multiple stressors, including a new job, that would require support and help from a clinician. The resident determines that a course of medication would be useful but that supportive therapy might be a useful addition.

Another thought is that the patient would benefit from seeing a therapist for at least 2 years. If the resident is about to graduate or switch to another clinical post, it might be in the patient's best interest to be seen by someone who can provide more long-term care.

The patient might say that he is unsure whether or not he wants psychotherapy and to make a commitment to be seen regularly for such treatment. In this situation, the resident might want to make sure that the medication is prescribed and will make the recommendation for another therapist to see the patient. Or the patient might live a distance from the university or hospital and is willing to come for the medical care but is not quite sure regarding the psychotherapy.

> **Competency:** The psychiatry resident must be able to determine under what conditions split treatment would be most appropriate for a patient and be able to convey these issues to the patient.

Scenario B

The patient has a strong bond with a therapist, who has referred the patient for medication. It is important at this point to obtain a separate explanation from the therapist of the reason for the referral. It could be that the patient has a perception that medication is needed. The therapist may feel that the treatment has reached an impasse—the patient is not doing well and is suggesting medication as a possible solution. It is critically important for the resident to have a conversation with the referring therapist, preferably before evaluating the patient, so that it is clear what the nature of the referral is and so that the expectations of the therapist are understood.

The resident must also understand what the patient is expecting from the evaluation. Is there an expectation that a pill will be prescribed? If not, what would that mean? The resident must perform a complete psychiatric evaluation and not make any assumptions about the diagnosis, history, or treatment. This evaluation must be conducted as if it were a de novo evaluation, even if there has been a discussion with the referring therapist. The resident must hear the story from the patient, including all the ingredients of a good evaluation: present illness, past psychiatric and medical history, family history, social history, review of systems, mental status, formulation, etc.

The resident needs to understand the expectations coming from the patient, the referring therapist, and anyone else—family members, friends of the patient—regarding why the patient is being seen for a psychiatric evaluation. It may be that the resident needs to speak with the patient's family doctor or other medical specialist and obtain laboratory studies, recent psychiatric or medical inpatient records, or other information before determining a treatment plan and course of action. It might be that the resident will need to call or speak to the referring therapist about the diagnosis and treatment plan before deciding on a course of action, especially when there needs to be a decision about use of benefits and sessions.

In certain situations, the resident might determine that it would be more helpful to take over both the psychotherapy and medication for a period of time, and when things are clarified and more stable, the patient could go back to the referring therapist. This kind of decision would have to be made carefully, with considerable attention being given to the transference and countertransference issues for the patient and the referring therapist. The resident must also have certainty about the reasons for this type of decision.

> **Competency:** The psychiatry resident should be able to demonstrate the ability to determine his or her role in a split-treatment arrangement and to obtain the appropriate information from the patient, medical records, the referring therapist, other medical clinicians, family members, and other sources.

Scenario C

In this scenario the patient has already been treated psychopharmacologically by another physician and is not doing well. Therefore, certain expectations have developed in the patient (and perhaps in the referring physician and therapist) about what the resident will be able to accomplish. At the beginning, it is important for the resident to talk with the referring physician and the therapist to better understand what has been tried pharmacologically, what type of psychotherapy has been provided, the sequence of the medication and the psychotherapy, any improvement in symptoms, other medical problems and medications, etc. Written documentation from the referring physician, including medication logs (including dosages, symptoms, and refills), is important. This will help the resident to review how long a medication trial lasted; whether the patient adhered to the trial regimen; how often medications were changed or combined; how often the patient was seen; and whether medication was monitored with visits, telephone calls, etc.

It is also very important for the resident to review all the medications with the patient, once again going over symptom changes, what made things worse or better, and any other factors that might have had an impact on the patient's use of the medication. Sometimes it is also helpful, with the patient's consent, to bring a family member in for part of a session to go over his or her assessment of the patient's symptoms when taking medications. The family member will often have a different perception of the various issues surrounding medications. This also provides the resident an opportunity to hear what other family members think of psychotropic medication and how they feel it affects the patient.

It might take a while to get all the information from the referring doctor, the therapist, the patient, and the family member, but the resident should not feel impelled to pick up the prescription pad at the first or even second session. In this scenario, the patient has not had as good a recovery as either the patient, the family, the doctor, or the therapist expected, so it is important to be as careful and thoughtful as possible.

An important question that needs to be asked by the resident in this scenario is whether the diagnosis that the referring doctor and therapist are using as the basis for medicating the patient is the correct one. Often, on closer review, there needs to be a change in the working diagnosis. Sometimes there is a substance use problem that was not previously uncovered. There could be an underlying personality disorder that was not previously understood that may be affecting the Axis I diagnosis. The patient may have developed a new medical condition or may have added a new medication, over-the-counter supplement, or alternative medication that is negatively affecting the patient's presentation of psychiatric symptoms. Or there could be new stressors, new pressures, a new relationship, or financial difficulties that the patient had not thought about bringing to the attention of the referring doctor or therapist that are clearly germane to the current symptoms.

Competency: The psychiatry resident should develop the ability to potentially reformulate a case.

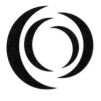

Evaluation and Opening in Split Treatment

In this chapter, we review the initial evaluation and opening of the treatment process of pharmacotherapy by a psychiatrist either 1) with a new patient who was referred to the psychiatrist by a nonmedical therapist or primary care physician for pharmacotherapy *while* the patient remains in therapy with the nonmedical therapist, or 2) with a new patient evaluated by the psychiatrist when the psychiatrist decides that this patient requires, besides pharmacotherapy, psychotherapy that will not be provided by the psychiatrist for various reasons (time constraints; economic reasons, e.g., the third-party payer does not reimburse for psychotherapy provided by a psychiatrist; or lack of expertise in a specific area or with a specific population, geographic area, etc.). We address the initial evaluation and related competencies in each of these situations. There are of course many other combinations and permutations, but we believe these to be two of the major types of situations that must be understood by residents.

The reader should be aware that parts of this chapter are taken directly from Chapter 3, "Evaluation and Opening in Integrated Treatment." The initial evaluations in integrated treatment and split treatment bear many similarities, but there are specificities that are important to point out and address. To make the point again, split treatment is also often called *collaborative treatment*, and some writers make a distinction that split treatment is not necessarily collaborative, in that the psychiatrist or primary care physician does not necessarily "collaborate" with the nonmedical therapist. Our view is that all care should be collaborative and that if the psychiatrist or other physician is not collaborating in some way with the nonmedical therapist, this is not optimal split treatment.

Initial Evaluation

As we note in Part I, "Integrated Treatment," the initial evaluation of any patient starts during the initial contact with the patient, whether this occurs over the telephone with a managed care intermediary, with a nurse who is collecting information, with a receptionist, etc. The patient begins to form an opinion and gets ready to develop or (not develop) an alliance with the clinician based on a myriad of events that begin before the first visit with the clinician.

The initial evaluation is mainly about collecting the data that the psychiatrist considers pertinent for making the diagnosis and deciding about the treatment plan—in this case, usually pharmacotherapy. Again, it should not be forgotten that the initial evaluation is also about forming the therapeutic alliance.

The referral for pharmacotherapy could be initiated by a nonmedical therapist who is well known to the evaluating psychiatrist and who could be closely collaborating with the psychiatrist (a preferable situation— truly collaborative treatment). This situation occurs frequently in residency training programs where residents get referrals for pharmacotherapy from nonmedical therapist faculty members, staff members, or trainees (e.g., psychologists, social workers, psychology interns).

However, the request for the initial evaluation and subsequent pharmacotherapy may be initiated by a nonmedical therapist not known to the resident or as a self-referral by the patient. We would like to emphasize that no matter who the referral source is and under what circumstances the referral was made, the initial evaluation should be the same: very thorough and detailed. Nothing should be left unexplored just because this information had already been obtained by the referral source and provided to the evaluating resident. The information from the referral source (if there is one) should be probed and checked with the patient. Accepting the interpretation of others could be misleading at times. Reinterpretation of clinical data using newly collected information could be very useful, helpful, and frequently essential for pharmacotherapy planning.

We have frequently seen a written referral for pharmacotherapy with a very specific request, for example, "Please evaluate patient for initiation of treatment with a selective serotonin reuptake inhibitor." Such requests should be viewed with caution and carefully evaluated. A request from a nontherapist should be discussed with the patient. It should be clarified whether the patient understands and agrees with the request. It should also be made clear that the request will not be automatically honored. The resident should make sure the patient understands that the decision about initiating pharmacotherapy and the selection of specific pharmacotherapy will be based on the initial evaluation and on possible laboratory and other evaluations. The resident should also explain to the patient that the decision about pharmacotherapy will be made in the best interests of the patient and based on the resident's best expertise and professional opinion. Thus, the resident's task may include overcoming some resistance and preconceived ideas about which pharmacotherapy should be chosen and what pharmacotherapy should be like (e.g., a nonmedical therapist may suggest to the patient that all her patients have been doing well with some particular medication, whereas the patient's symptomatology may require medication with a different efficacy or tolerance profile). The initial evaluation also presents a good opportunity to determine whether the patient has any negative issues about being treated by a resident and to review what type of supervision will be given to the resident regarding the patient's care.

It should be made clear to the patient and to the referring therapist during or before the initial contact that the first session (or even a few sessions) will be devoted to an evaluation, and only after its completion will any decision about pharmacotherapy be made. Also, to avoid further misconceptions and false expectations, the resident should inform the patient or the therapist of the length of the initial evaluation (some therapists may tell patients that the resident will spend just a few minutes with them).

Bender and Messner (2003) suggest that framing the first session as a consultation and evaluation may have an important advantage. Both the patient and the psychiatrist can evaluate whether they are a good match and whether they feel comfortable working with each other. Both are given "the freedom to view the first meeting as an introduction without an obligation to continue" (Bender and Messner 2003, p. 17). Framing the first contact as a consultation is probably much easier in an outpatient setting. The concept of the first session (or sessions) being a consultation/ evaluation may be also very useful in starting the treatment of children or adolescents. There are more parties involved, such as one or both parents, and getting a good match is therefore more complicated.

Conceptualizing the initial evaluation as a consultation may also better reflect the reality of the initial evaluation. Nonmedical therapists mostly refer patients for initiation of pharmacotherapy, but in fact the foremost question of the referral is consultative: "Is pharmacotherapy indicated, and only if it is indicated, would you initiate and prescribe?" The question of whether pharmacotherapy is really indicated should always be carefully pondered. Nonmedical therapists may at times and for various reasons get stalled in therapy or might not know what else to do. They may refer the patient for pharmacotherapy as a last resort, but pharmacotherapy may not be the solution either. Countertransference may play a major role in the therapist's approach to getting another opinion or pharmacological consultation. Therefore, when after a careful initial evaluation the resident concludes that pharmacotherapy is not indicated, he or she should resist the pressure from the patient or the therapist and should refuse to initiate pharmacotherapy. At times, having a discussion with the nonmedical therapist and suggesting a different therapeutic approach or even a different psychotherapy might be more appropriate.

> **Competency:** The psychiatry resident must be able to understand the various dynamic and biological reasons for the request for a psychopharmacological consultation and be able to obtain the appropriate information to make an informed decision about the diagnosis and treatment plan.

The initial step in the evaluation in both situations—either with a patient who was referred or with a patient who is seen de novo and will be referred for psychotherapy to a nonmedical therapist—is establishing an accurate diagnosis. It is important to emphasize that although the diagnosis is an important element in treatment decision making, it is not the sole element. The diagnosis does not provide much information about the individual and about the individual's need and particular issues in treatment planning. There are other elements—such as the patient's previous response to treatment, symptoms (e.g., sleep disturbance, suicidality), cooperation or resistance, family history, support system, medical history, treatment with other medication, possible previous treatment experience, and value and belief system; and the physician's skills and orientation towards other treatment modalities—that may have a significant impact on treatment planning. Thus, information about all these and other factors should be gathered in the first session (or sessions) to help inform the decision about treatment. Much of this information could and should be included in the referral note or initial evaluation by the nonmedical therapist (when the patient is referred for an evaluation by a nonmedical therapist or by a primary care provider). Nevertheless, we emphasize that this information needs to be checked and probed again.

First Contact: Technical and Introductory Remarks

The first contact between the resident and the patient usually starts in the waiting area. After being triaged and being given an appointment, the patient arrives full of various expectations. The patient may be coming to see the resident with various preconceived ideas, and he may have unrealistic expectations. For example, the therapist may have referred the patient after a more or less unsuccessful course of therapy, or the patient may have some negative transference feelings that have built up during the course of therapy (e.g., "physicians are cold, uninterested, just pushing pills").

The first impression is quite important. The patient is probably wondering, "Who is this doctor? What is he going to ask? Are we going to get along?" The patient is probably feeling a bit uncomfortable in the waiting area and does not want anybody else to know that he is coming to see a psychiatrist. In this era of increased concerns about confidentiality, the resident needs to make sure that the patient's identity is protected. Therefore, calling the patient by his last name in the waiting area might be problematic, because it reveals his identity. The resident can call the patient by his first name; however, that may not fare well with some patients, especially older patients. Many experts (e.g., Bender and Messner 2003) therefore advise psychiatrists to simply identify the patient who is waiting, approach him and ask whether he is waiting to see this particular psychiatrist, and then invite the patient to follow or come in.

For the psychiatry resident, one of the most difficult aspects of split treatment is figuring out who is really in charge of the patient. The answer is clear: the physician is in charge of the patient. However, confusion can arise when the patient has had a long-standing relationship with a therapist and is coming to see the resident for a particular aspect of the care: medication. The resident wants to evaluate the patient, obtain a full history, and make an assessment, but the patient might not understand why the resident requires so much information. The patient may wonder why the resident cannot obtain the information by reading the medical record or talking to the therapist. The patient might not understand why it all has to be rehashed.

After taking the patient to the office and making him as comfortable as possible (the patient might not feel comfortable spending the entire session sitting in his coat), the resident should explain what is going to happen during the first session or two. It should be made clear approximately how long the session is going to last and what is expected to come out of it. One should be aware that this is the time when the formation of a working therapeutic alliance begins. As Bender and Messner (2003, p. 29) point out, the therapist should be responsive and not overbearing at this time (and at other times) and should be careful not to underdirect or overdirect the first session.

In the case of an evaluation in a split-treatment arrangement, especially when the patient is referred for the evaluation after having been seen by a therapist, some of the central questions that the patient and the resident need to address during the initial evaluation session (or sessions) are the following:

- Why is this evaluation being requested now?
- What is the patient expecting?
- What is the referring clinician expecting?
- What is the expected outcome of this evaluation?
- What are the goals of this session?
- What is the level of understanding of the patient?
- Does the resident have enough information to do a complete evaluation at this session? Will there need to be one or more follow-up sessions to complete the evaluation?
- What is the level of confidentiality between the patient and the resident? How much can be discussed or told to the referring therapist? What are the lines of communication between the psychiatrist and the therapist, and how frequently will they be used?
- What is the patient's diagnosis according to the resident? Is it similar to or different than the diagnosis provided by the referring therapist?
- Which mental health professional should be contacted for which problems? (The patient should be instructed to contact the psychiatrist regarding any issues related to medication and also for other clinical issues, such as feeling worse or being suicidal.)

These are just some of the complicated issues that the resident must think about even before seeing the patient.

> **Competency:** The psychiatry resident should be able to determine the multiple issues that need to be addressed in the initial evaluation of a patient being referred by an outside therapist or physician or as a self-referral.

The resident should be observant of the patient's behavior during the initial period of evaluation: does the patient seem anxious, avoid making eye contact, wring his hands, have tremors, or sit at the edge of the chair? It is also polite, appropriate, and practical to inform the patient that confidential notes will be taken during the information-gathering session, if this is the case. The patient's feelings about the psychiatrist's note taking during the session should also be explored. As MacKinnon and Yudofsky (1991, p. 10) note, some patients may resent the psychiatrist taking *no* notes during the interview, because it would make them feel that what they said was not sufficiently important or that the doctor was uninterested. Other patients, as MacKinnon and Yudofsky also noted, cannot tolerate note taking because they feel that it distracts the psychiatrist's attention from them.

It is also important to make sure that writing information down does not become the dominant activity of the information-gathering session. One should write the basic information and scribble down the most important data without interrupting the flow of the interview and without avoiding or diminishing eye contact with the patient. There may also be times during the interview when the resident should stop writing notes, putting the pen and paper down. This applies to situations when intimate or sensitive issues, such as sexual issues or negative feelings about any previous treatment and therapist or physician, are discussed (MacKinnon and Yudofsky 1991).

In these times when nearly everything is computerized, many psychiatrists are switching to electronic medical records. The same rules applicable to paper writing apply to typing electronic notes. We advise psychiatrists not to type into the computer during the session. Paper notes could be transferred into the computer after the session. It is also advisable to transcribe or type notes right away after seeing the patient and not wait till the end of a busy day, when the memories of several patient histories could merge and facts could become confused.

Many psychiatrists start the initial evaluation by obtaining basic patient data such as age, marital status, and employment. Others advocate beginning the session with an open-ended question such as "Why are you coming to see me?"; "What can I do for you?"; "How can I help you?"; or, when the patient has been referred by a nonmedical therapist, "What is your understanding of why you have been sent to see me?" At times a further explanatory comment might be helpful, such as "I understand that you were referred to me by your therapist, but what I am interested in is why you originally went to see your therapist and what has happened since then." The patient should be left to answer this question without interruption if possible (although patients with mania, psychosis, or cognitive difficulties may have to be interrupted). The resident should acknowledge that he or she is listening by occasionally making comments or sounds such as "Hmm" or "Yes." The patient should be asked to provide more details whenever possible and appropriate. The psychiatrist should encourage the patient by making comments such as "Tell me more about this" whenever appropriate. One should also think and frame questions in terms such as "Why now; why at this point in the patient's life, is she coming to see me and telling me this?"

Although we discuss the information gathering in a certain structural fashion, progressing from the chief complaint and present illness through various parts of the history to the mental status examination, it is important to realize that 1) there are many overlaps between various parts of the examination (e.g., present illness and parts of the mental status examination); 2) the sequence of the patient evaluation is not engraved in stone; and 3) the resident should not avoid following cues for the sake of keeping to a rigid information-gathering outline. One mistake that is frequently made by beginning clinicians is putting aside certain matters that are seemingly unrelated to the questions asked. This could lead to missing a very important therapeutic issue, and it could also make the patient feel that the resident is not really interested in his or her concerns.

The initial evaluation is usually finished in a preliminary form within the first hour or so designated for the assessment. Evaluation of an inpatient (but not in the emergency department) may require more time. Often even the most experienced clinician may not be able to finish the initial evaluation and establish a preliminary diagnosis within the time frame of the first contact, and a subsequent evaluation session may have to be scheduled. Most initial evaluations of adult patients include evaluation of the patient himself or herself. The evaluation, however, may involve an interview of relatives or significant others in some cases. An evaluation of a child or adolescent should always, if possible, include an interview of parents or guardians (together with the child and also separately).

The resident and the residency training director must make sure that the clinic provides at least 1 hour to see a new patient for a psychiatric evaluation. Some clinics provide only 30 minutes, based on the assumption that an evaluation has already been performed by some other clinician. Thirty minutes is not adequate for any initial evaluation. There is too much information to gather, and the most important aspect of this evaluation, forming a therapeutic alliance, is very difficult when the patient already has an alliance with another clinician or therapist. Thirty minutes is too short a time even for an experienced clinician and is certainly not enough time for a resident at any stage of training. In addition, the discussion of prescribed medication and documentation takes a significant amount of time. If a patient is already in a split-treatment arrangement with a resident and the resident is making a transition off the service, the incoming resident should ideally see the patient for 1 hour for a new evaluation. The patient should not be charged for this new evaluation; it should be billed as a follow-up. This provides continuity, provides the resident with the opportunity to appropriately treat and learn about the patient, and does not encumber the patient with an expense because of the nature of the teaching service. The resident also must not be asked to do too many of these types of initial evaluations. Because these evaluations are so complicated and take so much time (both in the session and outside the session), much of which is not billable, it is very important to understand the limits of taking on such complex and time-consuming patients.

Furthermore, it is important for the resident to have an opportunity to receive supervision after seeing the patient and developing a formulation, not just during the initial evaluation. Many university clinics have an attending psychiatrist sit in on the evaluation session for key portions of the case. However, that may not really provide adequate time and setting for the resident to digest the information, think about the formulation and treatment plan, and be able to provide psychoeducation to the patient. In such settings it may be necessary either to ask the patient to leave the office for a few minutes or to have the resident and supervisor leave the office to discuss the diagnosis and treatment plan for a few minutes. However, such an arrangement may trigger transferential feelings and prompt the patient to wonder who is in charge. We have had good experience with residents briefly discussing the case and its disposition with the supervisor at the end of the evaluation in the supervisor's office (not in the hallway) and later discussing the case in more detail in case conference with the supervisor and ideally with another clinical or psychotherapy supervisor.

Although time may be viewed as a luxury, it is also something that is very necessary. It is important to be able to see the patient on another day, not just on the day of evaluation, and to determine whether the patient appears to be the same or different; whether some of the presenting symptoms remain or are changed; and—a key question—whether the patient returns for the follow-up. The resident must not make the mistake of prematurely reaching closure on a patient's formulation, diagnosis, and treatment plan. Providing the wrong medication or making the wrong diagnostic assessment can set the patient back for a long time; can have a negative impact on the therapeutic alliance between the patient and the resident (and future clinicians); and can potentially cause morbidity (or even death) in the patient. If a prescription is provided to a patient at the first session and the patient does not return for follow-up, this could add to potential liability and problems for the resident and clinic.

> **Competency:** The psychiatry resident must be able to balance the number of patients in split treatment with the complex and time-consuming nature of evaluating and treating such patients.

One of the ways to address the points outlined above is to begin to educate the patient about why it is so complicated to conduct an evaluation—not that the patient is so sick or difficult, which is what the patient might be worried about, but rather that it will take a while to do a thorough job, and that is what the resident wants to do. Most patients can appreciate that prescribing medication, making sure of side effects and drug interactions, taking age issues into consideration, and evaluating the effects of other medical problems all complicate the picture and that hastily prescribing medication and seeing if it works is not in the best interest of either the patient or the doctor. On the contrary side, some patients might think that the resident is trying to extend or drag out the evaluation to make more money, or that the resident is a trainee and is therefore not experienced, and therefore the resident must address these kinds of issues and thoughts.

Just like in integrated treatment, the resident must evaluate the patient and feel ownership of his or her care. Because others are involved in the care, the resident may sometimes feel like an intruder or a consultant with regard to the case. Although these are honest feelings, the physician is usually the key person if there is an untoward or untimely death or suicide or adverse outcome, so one of the key issues in the evaluation is for the resident to feel some ownership of the care of the patient (MacBeth 1999). There must not be a tug-of-war with the patient being in the middle. The therapist is asking for help, and the resident may be able to give it to the therapist and the patient. But the triangulated relationship is complicated by the question of who is in charge. Some would say that the patient is ultimately in charge. From a medicolegal standpoint, it is probably best for the resident to think of himself or herself as being in charge, even though there is at least one other clinician involved (MacBeth 1999). What follows then is thinking of the answer to the question, "In charge of what?"

> **Competency:** The resident must be able to articulate and understand his or her role in the split-treatment arrangement: responsibilities, structure, and liabilities.

This is where split treatment gets very complicated for the resident. There is considerable pressure on the resident to obtain all aspects of the patient's psychiatric and medical history, but the resident must then fragment off a portion of that history (usually medication management) while always needing to consider the whole patient, especially in relation to potential for suicide and violence, family issues, medical problems, etc.

While conducting the evaluation, the resident will be interested in all aspects of the patient, but then the resident has to determine how to convey to the patient that although certain characteristics will be focused on, the resident remains interested in and concerned about all aspects. Similarly, the resident needs to provide the patient with guidelines about when to contact the resident and how to inform the resident of changes in medical issues and other adverse events that may or may not be related to medication—in other words, helping the patient understand what should be ascribed to the medication and the medical aspects of care and what the patient should do if a situation arises that is not clear. Many such situations could occur, so the resident must communicate this information clearly in the initial evaluation.

Initial Evaluation Outline

The initial psychiatric evaluation should be fairly similar if not identical in any treatment arrangement discussed in this book: integrated, or split *after* referral from a nonmedical therapist or primary care physician, or split *before* referral to a nonmedical therapist or primary care physician. Initial evaluation after a referral from a nonmedical therapist may be somewhat modified and more difficult.

This evaluation is colored by information from the referring nonmedical therapist or primary care physician. Ideally, the entire chart is available and the resident has had time to read the referring note and at least skim through the chart. The evaluation in this situation could be more difficult because of patient transference and resistance to yet another long evaluation. Patients will also unavoidably compare the style and comfort level of the resident with those of the therapist. We emphasize again that it is essential to explain to the patient that the evaluation is going to cover many if not all of the issues (and probably more) that were already discussed in the evaluation with the nonmedical therapist and that the reasons for this are that 1) the psychiatrist wants to get a full understanding and picture of the case, and 2) because this evaluation is about medication treatment, some issues might not been covered in the evaluation by the nonmedical therapist.

In the sections that follow we point out the specific issues pertinent to an initial evaluation in split treatment after a referral from a nonmedical therapist. Otherwise, the initial evaluation is the same as in integrated treatment.

It is important to note that the order of various parts of the initial evaluation may be a matter of personal preference or custom. However, after obtaining basic identifying data, one should start with the inquiry about the chief complaint and present illness.

Chief Complaint and Present Illness

Even though the chief complaint is traditionally listed on outlines and forms of psychiatric evaluations, it is not something one always asks about, but rather identifies in the written summary of the examination. It could be a direct quote of the patient's response to the question, "How can I help you?" or "Why do you think you need help?" Or it could be a very brief, simple summary of the patient's main complaint ("Patient has been depressed for the past 3 weeks," or "Sudden onset of panic attacks 3 weeks ago"). It may also serve as an introduction to the next part of the evaluation: the present illness. In the split-treatment situation, the outlining of the chief complaint may just repeat the referring clinician's reason for referral (e.g., "The patient was referred for long-standing depression resistant to cognitive-behavioral therapy," or "The patient was referred for a sudden change in behavior and hearing voices during the course of dynamic psychotherapy").

The questioning about the history of the present illness should start with open-ended questions. These broad questions, however, should be replaced—depending on the clinical situation—by focused or targeted specific questions about the symptoms, their onset, possible precipitating factors, impact on functioning, the scope of distress, maladaptive patterns, and other issues. Some patients may be able to provide a fairly chronological account of their present illness. Others may need to be asked specific questions about the onset and other clinical factors. Depending on the clinical material provided by the patient, one may ask questions that may later help in the treatment selection (medication, psychotherapy, or both). The questioning usually becomes more direct and targeted through the interview. It may not always be possible to clearly separate the history of the present illness from the past psychiatric history or history of previous psychiatric illnesses. The history of the present illness could include what some call the psychiatric review of systems (MacKinnon and Yudofsky 1991). This review includes questions about the patient's sleep pattern, appetite, weight regulation, bowel functioning, and sexual functioning (MacKinnon and Yudofsky 1991). Assessment of suicidality should be also included in this part of the evaluation. Assessment of suicidality could start with broader questions such as asking whether the patient has been feeling that life is not worth living. The assessment of suicidality and homicidality, however, should ultimately be specific and well documented. (Does the patient have vague suicidal ideation or a specific plan? If the patient has a plan, is the selected modality available? What is the overall risk? Is a safety net available?) Just as in many other areas of questioning, when inquiring about suicidality or homicidality, the resident can mention the referral from the nonmedical therapist with a remark such as "Your therapist related to me that you were feeling like killing yourself." However, using the information obtained from the referring clinician must be done judiciously and carefully. At times the patient may not corroborate this information for various reasons (e.g., no longer feeling suicidal, being afraid of hospitalization, or not trusting the psychiatrist), and pressing the issue could lead to serious transference and resistance.

The interviewer should not remain focused on only one area of the problem and psychopathology. After establishing a very preliminary possible diagnosis, one should always probe other areas of psychopathology (e.g., in depressed patients one asks about anxiety, psychosis, etc.).

Psychiatric and Medical Illness History

The patient's history of psychiatric illness is a very important part of the initial evaluation. Such a history could have a tremendous impact on treatment planning and selection of treatment modality. A patient with a recent episode of major depression and a history of two previous episodes of major depression should probably start lifelong treatment of this illness. The suicidality of a patient with a history of several serious suicide attempts is going to be viewed much more seriously than a suicidal gesture in a patient with no previous history of suicidality. A positive response to previous treatment should guide one to use the same treatment again and vice versa—an unsuccessful treatment trial should guide one not to use the same modality again.

The patient should be probed about onset, possible precipitating factors, course, comorbidity, accompanying disability, and treatment. As noted above under "Chief Complaint and Present Illness," at times it is difficult to separate the history of the present illness and the overall psychiatric illness history. Information about psychiatric hospitalizations should include the patient's age at the time of hospitalization, reason for hospitalization, length of hospitalization, place of hospitalization (the psychiatrist may be familiar with the place and may need to obtain records from the hospital), what was done during the hospitalization (medications tried, psychotherapy), the patient's condition at discharge, and the patient's feelings about the hospitalization.

The patient should be asked about previously used treatment. Questions about medications should include the names of the medications, the patient's understanding of the reasons for using a particular medication, the length of treatment with each particular medication, maximum dosages, whether the medication was helpful, which symptoms were relieved the most, and what side effects were present. Questions about medication allergies should be also asked, but one should make a distinction between true allergy and a serious side effect. Many psychotic patients will frequently say that they are allergic to one of the antipsychotics. Detailed questioning may reveal that they had a dystonic reaction when taking a higher dosage. The patient should also be asked whether he or she is taking any psychotropic medication at the time of the initial evaluation. As Bender and Messner (2003) emphasize, one should not assume that the patient is not taking psychotropic medication if he or she is not seeing a psychiatrist. Many primary care physicians prescribe psychotropic medications. Many primary care physicians are even mandated by managed care companies to try psychotropic medication and to refer the patient to a psychiatrist only after the first treatment attempt fails. In the split-treatment arrangement it is quite important to probe the issue of previous use of medication. It has been our experience that nonmedical therapists frequently do not get a good medication history. Similar questions (when, why, what kind, success/failure, patient's feelings about the treatment) should be asked about previous psychotherapy and behavioral therapy. One should also ask whether medication was combined with psychotherapy or behavioral therapy in the past.

Previous suicidal thoughts and behavior should be explored and documented (age at the time of suicide attempt, relationship to symptoms, planned or impulsive attempt, modality used, feelings about death and dying at the time of the suicide attempt, whether it was a suicidal gesture, subsequent treatment, and the patient's current feelings about a particular suicide attempt). It is also important to make a distinction between suicidal and self-mutilatory behavior.

A thorough exploration of possible substance abuse history may be part of the overall psychiatric history or part of the personal and social history. The patient should be asked about substances abused (specific substances could be mentioned), age at commencement of substance abuse, duration (if not continuous), frequency, amount used, money spent for substance abuse, how the substance was obtained, possible association with illegal activities (e.g., selling drugs), complications (medical, e.g., hepatitis, acquired immune deficiency syndrome; psychiatric, e.g., depression, withdrawal, blackouts; relational; financial; employment-related), immediate effect of the substance abused (feeling better, improved mood, relief of anxiety), personal feelings about substance abuse (feelings of guilt or shame), in what situation substance occurs (alone, with a group), and previous treatment and its results (inpatient, outpatient). Similar questions should be asked specifically about alcohol abuse. Patients should also be questioned about tobacco (smoking or chewing, and how much) and caffeine use (the number cups of coffee a day, the amount of other caffeinated beverages).

Medical history is an important part of the psychiatric evaluation. The history of serious illnesses, especially chronic ones, and surgeries should be obtained. The resident should consider whether the presenting symptoms are either a manifestation of the chronic illness, a reaction to the chronic illness, or not related to the illness. Specific questions should also be asked to determine the possibility of a seizure disorder or head injury. The patient should also be asked about medications used to treat any medical conditions. Preferably the patient should provide a list of these medications and dosages. Many medications can induce various symptoms—such as depression, anxiety, and fatigue—and thus mimic mental disorders. Many medications can also interfere with the metabolism of psychotropic agents.

Female patients should always be asked about their menstrual history, including the age at menarche, regularity of the cycle, possible menopause depending on age, use of contraceptives, and symptoms associated with menstruation (pain, cramping, changes of mood, irritability), including their possible alleviation with hormones and medications (e.g., antidepressants). Women of childbearing age should be questioned and possibly tested regarding the possibility of pregnancy before starting medication.

The medical history could also include a brief review of systems.

We would like to point out that, for fairly obvious reasons, a good medical history is usually not obtained by nonmedical therapists. Nonphysicians frequently document medical history by the use of a questionnaire, which may just list the names of a few diseases without including any time frame or treatment documentation. Therefore, residents need to conduct a very careful medical history for each patient and not rely on information provided by the referring clinician.

Family History

Information about a family history of psychiatric illness and responses to treatment could also have an impact on treatment selection and planning.

Family history should include the family history of psychiatric and medical illness and exploration of relationships within the family. Information about both parents should include their ages if living (or age at the time of death and cause of death), history of mental disorders, history of medical illnesses, medications used to treat any psychiatric illnesses, and responses to medications. The information about siblings should include their ages (and thus also the patient's birth order), presence of psychiatric illnesses, treatments, and responses to treatments. A history of psychiatric illness and treatment in members of the extended family (grandparents, aunts, uncles, cousins) should also be obtained. Besides asking about mental illness, we recommend asking specifically about substance abuse and suicide history in family members. Many people do not think about substance abuse or suicide in terms of mental illness. One should also explore the relationships within the family: how the patient gets along with his or her parents and siblings, whether there has been any violence within the family, and whether any abuse (physical or sexual) has occurred.

Personal and Social History

Personal and social history is the part of the evaluation that makes the psychiatric evaluation different from an ordinary medical evaluation. Physicians in other disciplines may ask about parts of the personal history but do not usually obtain the personal and social history in its entirety. This part of the evaluation may help the examining physician with treatment planning in terms of the patient's preferences, family and social support, financial situation, affordability of various treatments, and other factors involved in treatment planning. The personal and social history encompasses several areas, and the clinician should attempt to elicit a full picture of the patient and his or her life situation.

The personal history may start with the perinatal and developmental history. Information about the prenatal situation (family constellation, whether the parents wanted and planned to have this child, possible complications of pregnancy) and the patient's birth (premature, uncomplicated, forceps delivery, cesarean section, jaundice at birth, defect at birth, etc.) should be obtained. Many pieces of information that some recommend gathering—such as the parents' reaction to the patient's gender and selection of the patient's name (MacKinnon and Yudofsky 1991)—might not be realistically obtainable under the ever-present time pressure. Some trainees, however, may have the luxury of having enough time to obtain this kind of information. Further information about personal history should include, if time and situation permit, developmental milestones, relationships during childhood and adolescence, and emerging personality (shy, defiant, oppositional) during childhood and adolescence.

Educational history should include information regarding whether the patient graduated from high school (if not, why not and whether a General Educational Development (GED) diploma was obtained), college education, postgraduate education (versus current employment), and original educational plans and their fulfillment. The patient should be asked about any history of difficulties, academic or behavioral, at school.

Occupational history should include, if possible, information about all employment, duration, reason for termination or change, any difficulties at work, and possible exposure to dangerous substances. An important question to consider is whether the patient's employment is commensurate with his or her education level.

Military history should include the age when the patient was drafted or recruited, reasons for signing up (idealism, financial reasons, or risk and thrill seeking), length of service, and the nature of and reason for discharge. It should also include information about whether the patient experienced combat, sustained any injuries, underwent any disciplinary actions, and was exposed to substances of abuse during service.

Relational and marital history should include information about any sustained relationship in the patient's life. Inquiry should be made about the age when the patient got married, length of marriage or relationship, past conflicts and disagreements, and present relationship with the partner or spouse. If the patient is divorced, reasons for divorce should be discussed. Information about children—their ages, health, education, and patient's relationship with them—should also be gathered. When the patient presents relational or marital issues as the core of his or her problems, the relational and marital history can be expanded by asking about further issues such as areas of disagreement, who does what at home, management of family finances, and relationships with members of the extended family.

Sexual history should include information about psychosexual development, early sexuality, sexual orientation, age of first sexual contact or intercourse, frequency of sexual activity, ability to reach orgasm, any sexual dysfunction (low libido, erectile dysfunction, lack of lubrication, premature ejaculation, delayed orgasm, anorgasmia, painful orgasm), masturbation, and unusual sexual preferences. We have noted that psychiatry residents frequently omit the sexual history for various reasons, either being uncomfortable asking patients about sex or inappropriately worrying about offending patients by asking about sexual history. We would like to emphasize that when asked tactfully and in full confidentiality, patients do not usually feel offended by questions about their sexuality, and in fact appreciate that someone is asking about this often neglected subject.

Some (e.g., MacKinnon and Yudofsky 1991) also suggest asking about social relationships, friends, religious and cultural background, hobbies, and long-term plans as a part of personal history. Others (e.g., Bender and Messner 2003, p. 66) recommend obtaining an "adaptive history" by asking questions such as "What stresses have you overcome in the past?"; "How did you do it?"; "What are your personal strengths?"; and others.

Mental Status Examination

The mental status examination is a summary of the physician's observation and the patient's subjective reporting of various areas such as appearance, behavior, feelings, perception, thinking, and cognitive functioning. Most textbooks describe the mental status examination as a long list of categories to be examined at the end of the psychiatric evaluation. An experienced clinician, however, usually begins the mental status examination from the very beginning of the evaluation by observing the patient's appearance and behavior and registering symptoms the patient reports. The more formal mental status examination conducted at the end of the psychiatric evaluation should therefore address only areas not previously covered, or areas in need of further clarification. One should not repeat detailed questioning about all symptoms of major depression in a patient who presented with a chief complaint of depressed mood, low energy, poor sleep, and lack of appetite. One might, however, ask about symptoms not mentioned before, such as anhedonia or cognitive impairment. We would like to emphasize that in a split-treatment arrangement a complete, well-organized, and well-documented mental status examination by the psychiatrist may be the only *complete* mental status examination to be conducted, and therefore it is extremely important that it be well done and documented.

The mental status examination should include but not be limited to the following areas:

Attitude—Whether the patient comes into the office voluntarily or hesitantly; whether the patient is cooperative, friendly, and appropriate; whether he or she makes good or poor eye contact; and the nature of the patient's facial expression.

Appearance—The patient's hygiene, clothing, and special marks (e.g., tattoos).

Behavior and psychomotor activity—The nature of the patient's gait; whether he or she is restless, sits on the edge of the chair, is wringing the hands, has increased motor activity; whether the patient has abnormal movements, tics, dystonias, gesticulations, etc.

Speech—The quantity (e.g., talking all the time or answering only in monosyllabic words) and quality (errors, tone, rate of production, rhythm, etc.) of the patient's speech.

Affect, mood, and their appropriateness and stability (vs. lability)—The "vegetative" signs such as sleep (including dreams), appetite, and libido should also be explored. Exploration of this area should also include other symptoms of mood disorders such as possible anhedonia, energy level, and feelings of guilt. Finally, one should ask about recent suicidal or homicidal ideation and possible plans.

Anxiety and related symptoms—Obsessions, compulsions, panic attacks, social avoidance, phobias, flashbacks, and startled responses.

Perception—Illusions, hallucinations, and feelings of unreality and depersonalization.

Thinking—Form (e.g., flow of associations, blocking, tangentiality, circumstantiality) and content (e.g., suspiciousness, ideas of reference, thought insertion, delusions—systematized, vague, or isolated—and their content—paranoid or grandiose) of the patient's thought processes; also, in the case of mood disorders, congruency with mood.

Alertness and wakefulness.

Orientation—By time, place, person, and situation.

Concentration—Tested by simple tasks such as serial sevens or spelling certain words forward and backward.

Memory—Recent, intermediate, remote, possible confabulation. Short-term memory and concentration could be tested by asking the patient to remember three things and asking him or her to recall them in 5 minutes.

Estimate of general information and fund of knowledge—The patient's ability to provide information about recent events, big cities, famous people, or geography.

Estimate of intelligence—Average, below average, above average, or possible mental retardation.

Judgment—Operational and formal; estimated by asking about reactions to standard situations.

Abstraction—The patient's ability to abstract could be tested by asking him or her to interpret proverbs or by discussing similarities and differences.

Insight—The patient's awareness of his or her illness or situation. Impulse control and frustration tolerance.

> **Competency:** The psychiatry resident should be able to understand and perform a complete psychiatric evaluation of patients who are in split-treatment arrangements.

Formulation

After finishing the evaluation, the examining resident may briefly formulate the case for himself or herself, considering the key issues such as the patient's present illness, past and personal history, developmental issues, and ego strengths and defenses. The formulation, however, may be postponed until further information is gathered and any test results have been obtained. In a split-treatment arrangement, the formulation should primarily rely on the information obtained by the resident but should also include and take into account information provided by the nonmedical therapist.

Diagnosis

Diagnosis (or diagnoses) of the patient should be made using the multiaxial DSM diagnostic classification (American Psychiatric Association 2000). Many consider the multiaxial diagnosis cumbersome and insufficiently inclusive. However, it forces the clinician to consider various areas that may have an impact on treatment planning and treatment outcome: diagnosis of major mental disorder, possible personality disorder or its traits, intellectual impairment, the presence of physical illness possibly involved in the pathogenesis and possibly complicating the treatment planning and outcome, the presence of major stressors, and the level of functioning.

Diagnostic considerations might include decisions about further areas of possible exploration such as a physical examination, laboratory testing (either exploratory, such as thyroid testing in unexplained tiredness and low energy, or as a baseline before starting certain medications, such as liver enzyme testing before beginning certain antipsychotics; or blood urea nitrogen, creatinine, and thyroid tests before starting lithium), measurement of heart rate and blood pressure before starting some medications, ordering possible psychological testing (e.g., memory and other cognitive testing), ordering neurological examination and other special-ized diagnostic testing, and conducting further discussions with the refer-ring nonmedical therapist.

Treatment Planning

The entire initial evaluation is focused on establishing the diagnosis and selecting the most appropriate treatment—in the case of split treatment, selecting the most appropriate medication. Both the diagnosis and the treatment selection and plan should be thoroughly discussed with the patient at the end of the initial evaluation (see "Discussion With the Pa-tient/Opening" below). The treatment selection is a very complicated process, which includes (in no particular order of importance and not exclusively) diagnosis; comorbidity; the evidence-based medicine data; possible use of guidelines; consideration of target symptoms; previous treatment experience (both efficacy and side effects); dangerousness (suicidality); the patient's beliefs, possible illness denial, preferences, misconceptions, and expectations; the patient's level of functioning and impairment; the patient's personality traits or personality disorder; pos-sible nonadherence to the medication regimen; possible involvement of another specialist (e.g., a nutritionist in the case of an eating disorder); psychodynamic issues; consideration of possible side effects; the physi-cian's experience and skills; formation of the therapeutic alliance; cost of treatment; insurance regulations; availability of both patient and treating physician; physical location of treatment (inpatient, day treatment, out-patient); existence of a support network; and also market seductions and pressures (on both physician and patient, such as those produced by di-rect consumer advertisement).

The issues specific to split treatment include the patient's relationship with the nonmedical therapist, the nonmedical therapist's attitude to-ward and relationship with the evaluating psychiatrist, specific insurance regulations (some insurance companies do not allow the patient to be seen by both the psychiatrist and the therapist on the same day), sched-uling difficulties for some busy patients (which can result in an additional series of visits), the patient's conscious and unconscious comparison of the psychiatrist and the therapist, and even the gender and ethnicity of both treating parties (e.g., a female patient dealing with a rape issue in therapy with a female nonmedical therapist is referred to a male psychi-atrist).

Bender and Messner (2003) suggest organizing psychiatric diagnoses into two categories: 1) disorders with targetable symptoms that meet

DSM diagnostic criteria (e.g., mood disorders, anxiety disorders, substance abuse), and 2) conditions more closely linked to ongoing life stressors (relational problems, occupational problems, adjustment disorders, personality disorders). This distinction may seemingly help to make the decision about medication versus psychotherapy. Psychotherapy, however, is usually indicated in both categories, and medication could be indicated in either category or both categories. In many instances, the impairment of daily functioning may be a major factor in choosing medication. For instance, the physician may recommend starting cognitive-behavioral therapy in a case of major depressive disorder with mild or no functional impairment; however, he or she will recommend an antidepressant plus cognitive-behavioral therapy in the case of major depressive disorder with severe functional impairment. The decision about selecting psychotherapy could be either therapist-based (whatever psychotherapy is the therapist's area of expertise), diagnosis-based (cognitive-behavioral therapy for depression or in vivo desensitization for agoraphobia without a history of panic attacks), or outcome-based (whatever the goal of therapy is, whatever could be realistically achieved; Makover 2004).

Treatment planning by the resident in a split-treatment arrangement always includes decisions about medication. In many instances, impairment in daily functioning may be a major decision factor in choosing medication. In the situation where the patient was referred by a nonmedical therapist for medication treatment, the decision usually includes only medication (unless the evaluating psychiatrist feels that psychotherapy is not indicated or a different psychotherapy modality should be chosen). Medication is selected or not, selection and other issues are discussed (see "Discussion With the Patient/Opening" below), and the patient is referred back to the therapist to continue in therapy.

Residents should realize that a referral for medication therapy by a nonmedical therapist does not automatically mean that medication is indicated. At times no medication is indicated. The nonmedical therapist may be frustrated by a lack of progress in psychotherapy, unrecognized resistance, or other issues and may be looking for a "magic bullet" in the form of medication. If the resident feels that medication is not indicated, he or she should explain this to the patient and later on discuss it with the referring nonmedical therapist. The reasons for not prescribing medication should be carefully explained and explored during these discussions.

However, in a situation where the evaluating psychiatrist sees a patient who was referred by a nonmedical therapist or was self-referred and is not in psychotherapy, the decision may include medication or psychotherapy or both. Again, if the resident believes that medication is not indicated, she should explain why not and decline to prescribe. If the resident feels that, in addition to or instead of medication, psychotherapy is indicated and he or she has no time or is insufficiently qualified, the resident should refer the patient for psychotherapy to a therapist with whom he or she is familiar and who is qualified in the particular psychotherapy chosen. As noted, the decision about selecting psychotherapy could be either therapist based (whatever psychotherapy is the therapist's area of expertise), diagnosis based (cognitive-behavioral therapy for depression or in vivo desensitization for agoraphobia without a history of panic attacks), or outcome based (whatever the goal of therapy is, or whatever could be realistically achieved) (Makover 2004). The resident should contact the therapist to whom she is referring the patient.

Discussion With the Patient/Opening

Discussing the diagnosis and the treatment selection and plan with the patient is usually the last step of the initial evaluation (unless the evaluation needs to be extended beyond the first session).

The patient should be informed, in simple terms, regarding the diagnosis and what the diagnosis means in practical terms. He should be encouraged to ask questions about the diagnosis and the diagnostic process. Interestingly, many patients are quite relieved once the diagnosis is made and they have a term—a symbolic explanation—for their problems. The patient should be informed whether or not the resident agrees with the diagnosis made by the referring nonmedical therapist, and if not, why not.

After discussing the diagnosis, the resident should briefly outline the initial treatment plan. In both kinds of split-treatment arrangements (either a patient referred by a therapist or a totally new patient), the resident should explain the selection of both the medication, what to expect of each modality, the time frame (e.g., fairly quick alleviation of anxiety with benzodiazepines vs. 3 weeks waiting for an antidepressant to alleviate depressed mood), and possible side effects and their management. The patient should be also given instructions on how to reach the resident in case there is an emergency or if the patient experiences any bothersome side effects or has any questions. It should be emphasized to the patient that she should primarily contact the resident about any issues related to medication or change in clinical status (especially suicidality or homicidality). Patients especially appreciate the possibility of such contact, and the availability of the resident often alleviates a lot of their anxiety about starting treatment.

The patient should be also informed that medication changes *could* be initiated between appointments over the telephone if necessary (e.g., in case of severely bothersome side effects). As with the diagnosis, patients should be encouraged to ask questions about the treatment. Many patients may have very specific questions based on their Internet searches, direct consumer advertisement, or media reports or sensationalism. Finally, the patient should be given a follow-up appointment fairly soon (it is simply not acceptable to say, "Here is your prescription; see me in month or two"), even if he sees his therapist somewhat frequently. Patients should be seen fairly often during the initial phase of treatment with medication. Providing medication fact sheets with specific information about side effects is often helpful to patients, so these should be available if possible. Some institutions and states require consent forms to be signed by patients or guardians when prescribing psychotropic mediations.

If the resident decides that medication is not indicated, he needs to discuss it with the patient very carefully and explain the reasons to the patient. Some patients will be relieved, because they are afraid to take medication. Other patients may get angry, because they expected (as the therapist did) a "magic bullet," which may not exist in their specific case, and they may feel as if the session with the resident was a waste of time and money.

If the patient is referred for therapy while being started on medication, the reasons should be explained to him or her (lack of time, insurance regulation, or lack of expertise by the resident).

As Beitman and colleagues (2003, p. 38) explain, the initiation of treatment should also include summarizing the patient's conceptualization of the illness and expectations of treatment, predicting possible side effects of pharmacotherapy, acknowledging negative treatment experiences, addressing the patient's denial of illness or need for treatment with inquiry into negative social consequences or lifestyle, and, in the case of pharmacotherapy, comparing mental illness and psychopharmacology to other medical problems and drugs, such as diabetes and insulin.

The subsequent sessions during the opening phase of treatment may further deal with issues such as the meaning of medication, fear of addiction to medication, loss of control over behavior, loss of personality, confusion of symptoms and side effects, the natural tendency to stop treatment when symptoms improve, and benefits and drawbacks of treatment (Beitman et al. 2003).

Pruett and Martin (2003) suggest other issues one should be aware of when prescribing medication and combining it with psychotherapy, such as the following:

- The clinician should be constantly aware of the seductions of marketing.
- Psychodynamic formulations are not a luxury but are necessary for making good treatment choices and for evaluating and reevaluating (on an ongoing basis) drug choice and the effectiveness of combined treatment.
- Psychiatrists should not be intimidated by time pressures, especially in the early appointments.
- Discussions of chemical imbalances are generally less helpful than many clinicians think, because it is so difficult to predict what they will mean to any given patient.
- The clinician should neither oversell nor undersell any one drug as a part of the treatment regimen but should instead tell the patient that there are other choices.
- **Psychiatrists should treat their patients as though the therapeutic relationship matters more than the pills—because it usually does.**

Once the initial evaluation—in one or more sessions—is completed, all information is gathered, and various treatment issues mentioned in this chapter are considered, the trainee should discuss the case with the clinical supervisor again.

The final part of the initial evaluation should be the contact with the referring nonmedical therapist or primary care physician or with the nonmedical therapist to whom the patient is referred to by the resident. These contacts should be arranged only with the patient's explicit agreement. Many institutions require written documentation of the patient's agreement. Some places have specific forms permitting such contact. The patient should not only be informed that this contact is going to happen but should also have some ideas of what will be discussed and whether this will be just a one-time contact (ideally it will not be) or a long-term arrangement.

The resident may contact the referring therapist or the therapist to whom she refers the patient in a letter or a written note (sent by regular mail or e-mail); however, personal or telephone contact is preferable. It should be noted in the patient's medical record that this communication occurred and the date and time.

In the case of contacting the therapist who referred the patient, the resident should thank the therapist for the referral and for the information provided. The resident's findings, diagnosis, and treatment decision, as well the treatment plan and further contacts between the resident and the therapist (who, when, in what situation, and why), should be discussed. If medication is not indicated despite the therapist's request, the reasons for not prescribing medication should be carefully and politely discussed. However, residents should avoid making premature changes based on pressure from the therapist and, conversely, criticizing the therapist in any way or making premature suggestions about the therapy.

In the case of contacting the therapist to whom the resident is referring the patient, the resident should explain the reasons for the referral, her plans for medication treatment, further contacts between the psychiatrist and the therapist (who, when, in what situation, and why), what she thinks should be addressed in therapy, and her reasons for making the psychotherapy referral. Regardless of whether the referral is appropriate or not, this information will help the therapist to understand the case and plan for therapy.

References

American Psychiatric Association: Diagnostic and Statistical Manual of Mental Disorders, 4th Edition, Text Revision. Washington, DC, American Psychiatric Association, 2000

Beitman BD, Blinder BJ, Thase ME, et al: Integrating Psychotherapy and Pharmacotherapy: Dissolving the Mind-Brain Barrier. New York, WW Norton, 2003

Bender S, Messner E: Becoming a Therapist: What Do I Say, and Why? New York, Guilford, 2003

MacBeth JE: Divided treatment: legal implications and risks, in Psychopharmacology and Psychotherapy: A Collaborative Approach. Edited by Riba MB, Balon R. Washington, DC, American Psychiatric Press, 1999, pp 111–158

MacKinnon RA, Yudofsky SC: Principles of the Psychiatric Evaluation. Philadelphia, PA, JB Lippincott, 1991

Makover RB: Treatment Planning for Psychotherapists: A Practical Guide to Better Outcomes, 2nd Edition. Arlington, VA, American Psychiatric Publishing, 2004

Pruett KD, Martin S: Thinking about prescribing: the psychology of psychopharmacology, in Pediatric Psychopharmacology: Principles and Practice. Edited by Martin A, Scahill L, Charney DS, et al. New York, Oxford University Press, 2003, pp 417–425

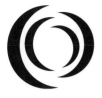

Sequencing and Maintenance in Split Treatment

Attempting to try to determine the best way to sequence psychopharmacology and psychotherapy in a split-treatment arrangement is a real and significant problem (Beitman et al. 2003). Although research has shown that the combination of both types of treatments are effective for patients with many kinds of psychiatric diagnoses, the research does not effectively lead to a guideline for sequencing. Furthermore, the guidelines that do exist based on certain types of disorders are focused on integrated treatment, in which a psychiatrist provides both the psychotherapy and medication management. Split treatment adds other variables that make the logistics and understanding of the sequence more complicated.

Along with the complicated nature of the sequencing, the other aspect is maintenance. Once the patient is stable with medications and some form of psychotherapy, some of the many questions to be addressed are how often the patient should be seen by each clinician; how often the medications should be changed; how often the family should be involved in the sequencing and maintenance phases; when termination should be discussed; and who should be managing the mental health benefit and completing the treatment plans.

It is also important to briefly note the historical backdrop regarding the sequencing of medication and psychotherapy, because it provides a context for the understanding of why this is so difficult. As Roose (2001) explains, there was a hierarchy in the analytic literature of first trying to treat patients with analytic treatment, which would be curative if effective. Medication was used only to relieve symptoms and could be used only if it would not affect the underlying psychic conflicts that were the origin of the psychological illness. Roose notes that in this context psychotropic medication was equated with inferior medical practice and it was believed that it could do significant harm if symptoms were masked enough that the psychiatrist could not determine, and therefore treat, the underlying psychic problems (diagnosis). Medications were to be used by inexperienced therapists and those who were not analytically trained—those who could not engage patients in a long-term dynamic relationship, where the real work would be taking place.

The psychodynamic community started to come around to the use of psychotropic medication when research began showing the positive effect of a combination of medication and psychotherapy (Rounsaville et al. 1981; Weissman et al. 1979). By the 1990s more analysts were reporting that they were prescribing psychotropic medications for their patients (Donovan and Roose 1995), but by 2000 it seemed that antidepressant medications were possibly still underprescribed by psychodynamic clinicians (Vaughn et al. 2000).

There is probably still a mind–body dualism—whether symptoms are biologically driven; whether patients have a chemical imbalance; whether some symptoms of anxiety and depression would eventually clear without medication; and whether some clinicians medicate too early or too late. These issues are all very important, and understanding the history of the field—realizing that some supervisors who are analysts were themselves trained under this mind–body dichotomy—is helpful to the resident and can promote greater understanding.

The resident is often further hindered by not necessarily always being involved in the care of the patient from the beginning—that is, from the point when the patient first entered the clinic for the psychiatric evaluation. The patient may be transferred from one resident to another for psychopharmacology, or the patient may have decided to end the psychotherapy with a therapist and is now coming to see the resident for medication. In either case, not knowing what was said at the beginning of the treatment, what the goals are and the expectations for care, and what the current resident is supposed to do vis-à-vis sequence are important questions.

In this chapter we raise the issues, questions, and problems regarding sequencing and then derive certain competencies that could be defined and measured.

What Comes First?

The first question, after performing a good evaluation, is to determine the diagnosis, or at least to have a working diagnostic formulation. Based on the diagnosis, an adequate treatment plan can be developed with consideration of medications or psychotherapy or both.

If the patient is already in psychotherapy with a clinician and is being referred for medication evaluation, then it is up to the resident to determine whether or not, on the particular day of the visit, he or she has enough information to consider providing medication. The most critical questions are the following:

- Does the resident need to get more information from the referring therapist or primary care physician?
- Does the resident have information about the patient's past and present medical history, current medications, and possible current pregnancy?
- Has consent about medication been obtained from the patient (and if the patient is a minor, from a guardian or parent)?
- Does the patient seem willing to take medication?
- Will the patient be able to have the prescription filled and pay for it, to be able to take the medication in a sustained manner?
- Will the patient be able to understand the instructions given regarding the benefits and risks of the medication?
- What are the consequences of not providing medication at this visit?
- When is the next time the patient will be able to return for a follow-up or call to provide feedback?
- Does a supervisor need to hear about the case before the resident prescribes? If this is not required, would it be better practice for the resident to obtain supervision?
- Is countertransference on the part of the referring therapist the reason for the referral for a medication evaluation? Is the patient or the therapist feeling frustrated about how the patient's symptoms are being handled in psychotherapy?

> **Competency:** The psychiatry resident should be able to gather enough information to safely prescribe medication.

If the patient is entering treatment for a psychiatric evaluation and the resident determines that the patient should see another clinician for psychotherapy (i.e., the patient will be in a split-treatment arrangement), the resident needs to determine whether to prescribe medication at this visit or wait until the patient has seen the other clinician. Furthermore, the resident needs to work on dynamic and other issues (e.g., transference) and determine whether these issues would affect the type and dosage of medication that would be used. It is also important for the resident to obtain answers to the following questions:

- Does the patient have certain symptoms (e.g., sleep disturbance) that may become worse while waiting for a another clinician to see the patient?
- Does the patient have a psychiatric diagnosis (e.g., schizophrenia, major depression) that would make the use of medication at the first visit seem more reasonable than not?
- Does the patient have a personal or family history that suggests medication would be quite useful?
- Does the patient have a preference or desire for (or on the contrary, a resistance to) starting medication at the first visit?
- Does the patient's home geography make it difficult to return for a follow-up visit in a short period of time, making it more important to think about medication at the first visit?
- What would be the impact of medication on patient's performance (work, etc.), and does the patient possibly need time off from work?
- Does the patient have a suicide risk, and if so, what is the plan for suicidal ideation and plan management?
- What is the patient's safety network?
- How much medication should be safely provided?

> **Competency:** The psychiatry resident should be able to determine the factors that might make it judicious to provide medication at the first visit.

Although the psychiatrist thinks of the patient as being in a split-treatment arrangement, in reality the patient is receiving collaborative treatment and should at least have the feeling that the care is integrated and unified. It is therefore important for the resident to understand that although there are at least two clinicians providing the psychiatric care, the patient should perceive the care as being seamless.

What Comes Next?

Assuming that the resident decides to provide medication to the patient at the first visit, what should follow is outlined below.

- The resident needs to determine what the major side effects of providing medication could be, what information regarding side effects should be given to the patient, and what the provision for management would be if side effects occur (e.g., should the patient call the resident or discontinue medication?). We recommend that the resident consider asking the patient to call the resident between the first and second appointments to relay how he or she is doing with the medication.
- The patient should be instructed to call the resident between psychiatric appointments if any changes occur regarding other medications or physical conditions (e.g., being prescribed a new antihypertensive medication).
- The resident should make sure that consent is obtained from the patient to send copies of the evaluation, including the medication information, to the referring clinician and other medical clinicians involved in the patient's care (e.g., cardiologist).
- Although all follow-up psychiatric notes do not necessarily have to go the outside clinicians (e.g., cardiologist) and therapist, the resident needs to have some regular communication with these clinicians regarding medical issues (such as medication and safety).
- If medications are prescribed, we recommend that the resident have the patient bring in a close significant other to a future meeting to discuss any issues the family member might have, especially regarding medication.
- Thorough medical records should be kept and should include what the resident has told the patient regarding side effects, time course of medication, etc.
- If there is such a requirement by the local or state authorities, the consent to take psychotropic medication should be completed and placed in the patient's chart
- The resident should ask the patient how best to prescribe the medication: for example, some patients send away for larger supplies to cut down on their copayment; some managed care companies require certain types and dosages of medication to be prescribed; some managed care companies require preauthorization of medications, particularly those that are not on the formulary.
- The resident should discuss whether any small children live in the home and how to keep the medication safely out of their reach.

> **Competency:** The psychiatry resi-
> dent should be able to demonstrate
> that appropriate members of the
> patient's clinical team will know
> what medical care and medications
> are being recommended or provid-
> ed by the resident.

What if Medication Is Not Prescribed?

If a therapist or other clinician refers the patient to the resident and the resident decides *not* to provide medication, what does this mean to the patient and the referring clinician?

There could be expectations on the part of the patient that medication is the answer to the patient's problems and symptoms. The patient could therefore be quite disappointed if the resident does not see the need to medicate. If there seems to be no basis for a biological etiology for the patient's symptoms, a different degree of responsibility might be placed on the patient for the current problems.

The patient might become angry that he had to pay for an evaluation that resulted in no treatment. It could be that the patient would value this type of evaluation only if it resulted in a prescription being given.

Based on what the resident observes in the initial appointment, he or she might disagree with the referring clinician's diagnosis. The resident might tell the patient that there does not seem to be a need for medication now but that judgment will be reserved until future sessions.

The patient might be pleased that medication is not being provided. The patient might not have wanted to take medication anyway (perhaps because he is frightened about taking them) and is relieved that it is not going to be prescribed. Furthermore, not having to take medication means that the cost of treatment will potentially be lower.

Family members or significant others might also have expectations about medications and what it means if the resident does not prescribe. They might have had strong hopes and expectations that medication would quickly provide major changes to the patient's problems, and these hopes are dashed when the resident does not prescribe.

Countertransference issues are often involved when a therapist recommends that a patient be seen for medication evaluation. Many questions about the situation may occur to the patient: Why is the evaluation being ordered at this time? What kinds of symptoms are frustrating for the therapist? Why can't the therapist fix the problems with psychotherapy alone? What does this mean with regard to the diagnosis? Was the therapist not doing a good enough job? Did the therapist miss something in the ongoing psychiatric care that led to the medication evaluation? What does it mean to get another clinician (the psychiatry resident) involved in the care?

The resident also has to make sure that she is getting supervision to best understand the dynamics of this complex situation. Often these types of split-treatment cases are not supervised by the long-term supervisor (who tends to supervise only one or two cases); the general outpatient supervisor tends to just go over the problem cases or the cases that the resident brings to his or her attention. These split cases are often overlooked in the supervision process because on the surface—because there is no medication involved—they seem to pose no problem. It is precisely these types of cases that are the most worrisome because of issues and questions that might have been overlooked in the interview, problems that the patient might have been masking, or the inexperience of the resident. We recommend that training programs assign supervisors expressly for the integrated or split-treatment cases to help residents to deal with the issues specific to these treatment arrangements.

If medication is not prescribed at the first session, the resident might ask the patient to come back in a few weeks for a reassessment. Often patients, like anyone else, present differently at different times. One could view this kind of arrangement as an extended evaluation or an evaluation with a follow-up. This gives the resident another chance to review the symptoms, think about the patient in the interim, and determine whether the original diagnosis and treatment plan should stand.

It also gives patients an opportunity to think about whether they want to return to see the resident, what it means to receive medication or not, and to talk about this issue with their therapist.

There is actually a great deal of pressure on the resident to get out the prescription pad and write a prescription for a patient at the initial visit. Under these circumstances it is probably easier to write a prescription than not to write one. It is therefore important for the resident not to feel pressured by the expectations of the patient, the family member, and the referring therapist if the resident does not feel that medication is indicated.

Competency: The psychiatry resident must determine when not to prescribe medication in a split-treatment arrangement.

If Medication Is Prescribed, How Often and What Kind of Collaborative Process Should Be Arranged for the Patient?

With any patient, once medication has been started it is usually a good idea to see the patient more often than usual until the psychiatric symptoms have stabilized and any untoward side effects can be minimized. This process might require that the patient be seen every 2–3 weeks or even more frequently at the beginning of pharmacotherapy. Telephone calls or e-mails between sessions can also be used. We recommend that the first follow-up visit take place within 1 week, if possible. Having frequent visits during the initial phase of treatment not only can be useful in the management of side effects but also can help in building the doctor–patient relationship and in overcoming the patient's disappointment with the delayed onset of action of some medications.

Because it is difficult to remember exactly what was said during the visit, it is important for the psychiatry resident to write down instructions for taking medications. Most emergency rooms and inpatient units provide written instructions for patients, as do many general medical and surgical clinics. It is a good idea for the resident either to type out the instructions about dosing, side effects, etc. for each patient or to have preprinted forms on which the pertinent instructions can be checked off. Some clinics have such forms available for use. This type of instruction should be made a routine part of each discharge.

It should be made clear to patients whom they should call when new symptoms develop. For example, if a patient starts to have suicidal feelings after beginning to take an antidepressant, should she call the therapist or the resident? We urge psychiatry residents to ask their patients to let them know when such feelings arise and also to convey to their therapist that the resident wants to be told about any suicidal, homicidal, or violent feelings that the patient has developed. When such symptoms develop, the patient should of course be seen promptly by a medical professional, which might include asking the patient to go an emergency room.

It is important to talk with patients about when certain symptoms might be alleviated (weeks vs. days) and what to expect if the symptoms are not relieved (perhaps increasing the dosage, changing the time of dosing, or changing medications).

It is a standard tenet in medicine to do one thing at a time so that the effect of the change on the condition can be observed. If the patient is already in psychotherapy or begins receiving psychotherapy at some point during the time medication is prescribed, then it is very hard to control for the effects of the medication versus the effect of the combined medication and psychotherapy. As Roose (2001, p. 45) notes, "there has been to date no systematic study of combining medication with psychodynamic psychotherapies." It is therefore almost impossible for the clinicians and the patient to determine the cause and effect of any changes or the full impact of either psychotherapy or medication when they are being combined. Therefore, the clinicians have to work very hard with each other and with the patient to try to determine if the combination is having an impact on the patient and whether the impact is positive or negative.

We have avoided referring to specific diagnoses; however, we need to point out that patients with borderline personality disorder or other Cluster B personality disorders could pose especially difficult situations in split treatment. As Gabbard (2001) points out, many patients with personality disorders are currently treated with a combination of medication and psychotherapy, although the scientific evidence is limited and most of this treatment is based on clinical impressions that patients with personality disorders have better outcomes with this combination than with either treatment modality alone. Various medications and therapies have been used and combined in patients with personality disorders, with the choices of medication frequently depending on the target symptoms (e.g., neuroleptics for the cognitive-perceptual symptoms; antidepressants for the affective and mood symptoms; and selective serotonin reuptake inhibitors, mood stabilizers, and other medications for impulsive-behavioral symptoms).

Combining treatment modalities is almost a rule in Cluster B personality disorders. These patients frequently end up in resident-staffed clinics and in split treatment. They pose a difficult management problem for residents in integrated treatment and especially in split treatment. In the split-treatment setting, many of these patients tend to play treaters against each other by disparaging one treater to the other. They may tend to idealize the prescribing physician and devalue the therapist, or vice versa (Gabbard 2001). In resident-staffed clinics, these patients may also idealize the *previous* prescribing resident (together or alone with the therapist) and demonize the resident who has just assumed their care. Such patients, for example, may demand more time for pharmacotherapy appointments, arguing that the therapist spends more time with them (or the previous resident spent more time with them) and cares more about them. As Gabbard illustrates, these patients might also demand that the omnipotent resident rescue them from the neglectful treatment by the nonprescribing therapist. This pattern of behavior is called *splitting*.

As Gabbard (2001) points out, this type of splitting is inherent to borderline personality disorder and cannot be entirely prevented or avoided. There are, however, several measures that could be taken to minimize the destructive impact of splitting on the treatment process. These measures should be made very clear to the patient at the beginning of both treatment modalities (pharmacotherapy and psychotherapy) and also whenever a new resident takes over the case.

The first measure is frequent communication and consultation between the treaters. The second measure is ensuring that certain limits specific to the case are established and discussed with both the patient and the treater at the onset of treatment (either—preferably—with all parties together, or with each separately). Examples are limiting the discussion of medication and side effects only to the medication reviews with the psychiatrist, or limiting the use of telephone calls or e-mails to each treater. Finally, as Gabbard (2001) suggests, both treaters should agree that "when the patient begins to disparage one of the treaters, the clinician who receives the information should contact the other treater to discuss what is going on rather than acting on the information given by the patient" (p. 89). If the patient does not agree with these rules up front, the resident should probably not agree to treat the patient (Gabbard 2001).

Although the split-treatment arrangement seems to provide a basis for splitting in patients with borderline personality disorder, this treatment arrangement may also provide some advantages for the treatment of borderline personality disorder. As Gabbard (2001) notes, in split treatment the intensity of transference may be diluted by having two treaters: the patient cannot avoid psychotherapeutic issues by focusing on medication (as could happen in integrated treatment), and treaters may gain insight from each other because they have different perspectives.

Making Changes

The psychiatry resident sees the patient at least every 2–3 weeks for medication adjustments while at the same time the patient is seeing another therapist for psychotherapy. It is very important that the resident and the clinician talk to one another to determine the impact of the medication on the psychotherapy. Is the patient staying engaged in the psychotherapy? Is the patient angry with the therapist over being sent to the psychiatry resident for medication? Does the patient feel annoyed about having to see two clinicians, paying for two clinicians' time, and worrying about whether there is communication between them? It is important that the patient does not become "monkey in the middle," that is, the communicator between the resident and the therapist. Communication between the resident and the therapist needs to be worked out at the beginning of care and could take place in person or by telephone, secure e-mail, fax, etc. The patient should be apprised of these communications and the method of communication.

In this kind of split arrangement, residents often feel pressured to make medication changes. If the patient is not being seen very often, the resident might be inclined to make changes (e.g., increase dosages, switch too quickly to another type of medication, or add a new medication to the regimen) whenever he or she sees the patient. If the resident starts feeling pressured to do this, he or she should consider seeing the patient more often or asking the patient to call between visits to talk about medication issues.

Maintenance

What constitutes maintenance in a split-treatment arrangement, especially when some of the symptoms are related to psychic conflicts? Is the alleviation of all symptoms the goal of medication?

At the beginning of treatment, it is important for the resident, the therapist, and the patient to determine the goal of medication to avoid undermedicating or overmedicating. If sleep is the target symptom, the goal of the medication might be to ensure that the patient is able to fall asleep in a reasonable time and to stay asleep in order not to feel somnolent during the day, to be able to work, etc. Similarly, if the goal is for the patient to have no depressive symptoms, then other aspects of the patient's life—such as employment or marital difficulties—might need to change before medications are changed.

Self-report measures, such as the Beck Depression Scale, are sometimes useful to permit patients to monitor themselves regularly and determine where they are on a symptom checklist. This helps give the patient and the clinician a reference point and allows them to talk about the specific issues that might be getting in the way of the full resolution of the patient's psychiatric problems.

During the maintenance phase, it is a good idea to talk about termination. What is the end point of the split treatment? The termination should be sequenced, with the medication and the psychotherapy being completed at separate times. The decision regarding termination should be a mutual agreement between the patient, the therapist, and the psychiatry resident.

If the resident is going to be rotating off the service or graduating, this is also considered a termination with the resident, although it is not necessarily a termination of treatment. Many junior residents do not appreciate the importance of their work with patients and therefore try to minimize the significance of the termination that comes with graduation. They may broach the issue just when they are about to leave without giving the patients enough warning. Or they might feel bad about leaving, as if they were abandoning their patients.

It is really important to try to match patients up with each resident and not just hand over an entire list of patients to the next resident. Patients want to know who they will be seeing and why they are being assigned to that particular resident. They want to know if there will be a proper signoff, if they will need to tell their entire story again to the next resident, etc. These terminations should be discussed during the maintenance phase, and proper time and attention must be paid to this important issue.

> **Competency:** The psychiatry resident should be able to demonstrate knowledge that the issues of maintenance in split treatment include termination issues.

The issues of termination are discussed in detail in Chapter 9, "Termination in Split Treatment."

Conclusion

Sequencing of pharmacotherapy and psychotherapy in split treatment is very difficult. Many patient variables, diagnostic issues, and communication patterns between the referring clinician and the therapist need to be worked out, and there are no clear guidelines based on research.

Furthermore, if multiple patients are being cared for in this kind of arrangement, there are often multiple therapists for the psychiatry resident to deal with. The task of working with so many clinicians is quite difficult and taxing.

We recommend that supervisors and training directors take particular heed of this last point. To the extent possible, we recommend that training programs not ask residents to have so many patients in split treatment with so many different therapists that the resident cannot develop a good working relationship with each therapist of every patient they see. Although we understand that this situation often occurs in private practice, it is neither optimal nor acceptable to place residents in such a difficult situation during training.

We also recommend that residents be provided good supervision on their split-treatment cases, especially during the beginning of each case, during maintenance, and when termination is discussed. It is hard for patients to terminate with their doctors, and inexperienced residents often do not appreciate or do not want to appreciate the strong transference feelings that patients develop, even in a short time, with residents nor the countertransferential feelings that the residents have engendered.

For this difficult subject it is also sometimes very useful to have ongoing group supervision of residents, using seminars structured around case conferences and clinical material to help incorporate the principles of both psychotherapy and pharmacotherapy.

References

Beitman BD, Blinder BJ, Thase ME, et al: The sequencing problem (using panic disorder as an example), in Integrating Psychotherapy and Pharmacotherapy: Dissolving the Mind-Brain Barrier. New York, WW Norton, 2003, pp 85–103

Donovan SJ, Roose SP: Medication use during psychoanalysis: a survey. J Clin Psychiatry 56:177–178, 1995

Gabbard GO: Combining medication with psychotherapy in the treatment of personality disorders, in Psychotherapy for Personality Disorders. Edited by Gunderson JG, Gabbard GO (Review of Psychiatry Series; Oldham JM and Riba MB, series eds.). Washington, DC, American Psychiatric Publishing, 2001, pp 65–94

Roose SP: Psychodynamic therapy and medication: can treatments in conflict be integrated? in Integrated Treatment of Psychiatric Disorders. Edited by Kay J (Review of Psychiatry Series; Oldham JM and Riba MB, series eds.). Washington, DC, American Psychiatric Publishing, 2001, pp 31–50

Rounsaville BJ, Klerman GL, Weissman MM: Do psychotherapy and pharmacotherapy of depression conflict? Empirical evidence from a clinical trial. Arch Gen Psychiatry 38:24–29, 1981

Vaughn SC, Marshall RD, MacKinnon RA, et al: Can we do psychoanalytic outcome research? A feasibility study. Int J Psychoanal 81:513–528, 2000

Weissman MM, Prusoff BA, DiMascio A, et al: The efficacy of drugs and psychotherapy in the treatment of acute depressive episodes. Am J Psychiatry 136:555–558, 1979

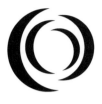

Termination in Split Treatment

In this chapter we review several scenarios for termination in split treatment. Because of the complexity of this kind of care, the scenarios cannot include every type of situation that might arise. Therefore we focus on some of the major termination issues so that the resident can achieve and sustain competency in this important and frequently encountered phase of clinical care.

Because termination of pharmacotherapy in split treatment bears some similarity to the termination of pharmacotherapy in integrated treatment, parts of the discussion of terminating pharmacotherapy are similar to the corresponding discussion in Chapter 5, "Termination in Integrated Treatment."

General Aspects of Termination in Split Treatment

Sequential or Simultaneous

In the split arrangement, treatment could be terminated either sequentially (initiating termination with either pharmacotherapy or psychotherapy) or, rarely, simultaneously (either after mutual agreement or, more frequently, forced unilaterally). The psychiatry resident is usually actively involved in terminating pharmacotherapy (while psychotherapy is either continuing or not). Nevertheless, this does not mean that the resident would not or should not be involved in dealing with issues surrounding the termination of psychotherapy by the nonmedical therapist.

The simultaneous termination of pharmacotherapy and psychotherapy occurs infrequently in split treatment. It could be forced by the patient's life circumstances (e.g., geographical relocation) or caused by the patient's withdrawal from treatment, either due to economic reasons (lack of money for treatment paid for out of pocket or a decision by the third-party payer that costs outweigh the benefits; Makover 2004) or due to the patient's feeling that treatment is no longer needed because he or she feels well.

Who Initiates Termination and When?

Patients might discuss the termination with both treating parties (psychiatrist and nonmedical therapist) or might just stop showing up for treatment. Patients who do not show up do not terminate, but quit treatment (Bender and Messner 2003). It is important to note that many clinics have a policy regarding no-shows. For example, patients must be called by telephone after missing an appointment for the first time. If no contact is made, a letter (sometimes certified or registered) is sent to the patient asking if he or she wants to continue treatment.

Termination is occasionally initiated by one or both of the clinicians, either because of the patient's nonadherence with treatment (rare for both treatment modalities) or because the patient has not paid for treatment. In general, a private psychiatrist does not have a legal duty to treat patients who are unable to pay (Simon 2004). However, private psychiatrists should be careful not to abandon patients (Simon 2004).

A special case of termination in split treatment occurs during residency training: some patients receiving pharmacotherapy from psychiatric residents may be transferred to another resident when the treating resident leaves the program, while psychotherapy with the nonmedical therapist continues. Although this is viewed as a transfer, it can also be viewed as termination from one resident and the beginning of treatment with another resident.

Termination of any treatment should always be planned well ahead, preferably several months in advance. The discussion and planning of termination may start from the very beginning of the treatment, as suggested by Makover (2004); however, such careful planning is rare. Besides careful planning, the success of termination depends on various other factors, such as the efficacy and outcome of collaborative treatment, the collaborative relationship with the nonmedical therapist, overall treatment goals, and financial resources. The supervisor has a key role in helping the resident to anticipate such termination issues.

Communication between treating parties is very important during termination. For one thing, thoughtful use of either psychotherapy or pharmacotherapy could be helpful in terminating the other form of therapy. Psychotherapy by the nonmedical therapist could be extremely helpful during termination of pharmacotherapy. It may help ease the patient's anxiety and help the patient adjust to life without medication. Termination of psychotherapy by the nonmedical therapist in split treatment could be helped or facilitated by continuing pharmacotherapy.

The resident should be aware that termination of either pharmacotherapy or psychotherapy is frequently difficult and may trigger strong transference and countertransference. The remaining treating party (either the psychiatrist or the nonmedical therapist) may be left to deal with unresolved issues between the patient and the other treating party, especially when termination is one-sided, forced either by the patient or by the treating party.

Pharmacotherapy or psychotherapy should be terminated after a mutual agreement and in collaboration with the patient. Termination should be discussed with the other treating party (i.e., the nonmedical therapist should be forewarned about pharmacotherapy termination by the psychiatrist and vice versa). As Beitman and colleagues (2003) note, there are several issues that both treating parties should be aware of: 1) clinicians need to respect both the patient and each other's professional understanding; 2) there must be an agreement that either clinician can terminate the split treatment but that the patient must be provided adequate and appropriate warning and referrals to other clinicians; and 3) both clinicians should preferably discuss how to stagger the termination (Beitman et al. 2003).

The decision about sequencing the termination (if both treatment modalities are planned to be terminated) should be discussed with both the patient and the other treating party, either together or separately.

> **Competency:** The psychiatry resident should be thinking about and anticipating aspects of termination throughout all phases of split treatment.

Terminating Pharmacotherapy First

Psychiatry residents will probably encounter the situation of terminating pharmacotherapy first more frequently—either they will be leaving the service or training program or they will terminate a successful course of pharmacotherapy (e.g., 6- to 9-month treatment of the first episode of major depression with an antidepressant, or 1-month treatment of acute job-related stress with a benzodiazepine).

The discussion of pharmacotherapy termination frequently starts at the beginning of pharmacotherapy. This discussion could be triggered by the patient's uneasiness about taking psychotropic medication. In the case of referral by a nonmedical therapist of a patient for pharmacotherapy, the patient might feel quite uncomfortable because he perceives (rightly or wrongly) that his illness or problem is becoming really serious. Besides asking about the side effects, one of the first questions many patients ask is, "How long will I have to take this medication?" The resident should provide an honest answer, including the possibility that he or she does not know or is not sure.

This discussion may be complicated by misconceptions or unwittingly false promises given to the patient by the nonmedical therapist. The therapist may try to ease the patient's anxieties by stating that the treatment is going to be quite short and easy. In cases when the patient initiates the referral for pharmacotherapy, the nonmedical therapist may, consciously or unconsciously, introduce some negative transference in the patient, either toward the medication or toward the psychiatrist (e.g., "You may never get off the medication"; "You will become dependent on the pill"; "You should not take it long so you don't become dependent on this crutch").

The initial discussion of treatment and formulation of the treatment plan should always include the goals and the best possible time for termination (Beitman et al. 2003). This discussion should be specific (as much as possible) and clear. For instance, specifying the duration of pharmacotherapy in case of the first episode of major depression is relatively easy. The patient should know that she will continue taking the antidepressant (at its full dosage) for 6–9 months after reaching remission, which in lay terms means after starting to feel and function well.

The issue of counting the duration of the continuation of pharmacotherapy from the time of feeling well is important. It can frequently take 2–3 months to reach full remission. Patients may start to press for termination of medication in another 3 months—clearly an insufficient time. This information should be also related to the nonmedical therapist so he or she can plan to include the termination of pharmacotherapy into the discussion during therapy sessions. The collaborating therapist should have a full understanding of the multiple issues and factors that are occurring in the course of termination of pharmacotherapy. An understanding, involved, and informed therapist could be extremely helpful in terminating pharmacotherapy in split-treatment arrangements.

The suggested length of pharmacotherapy varies from disorder to disorder and depends on various factors (chronicity, severity, and recurrence of the disorder; previous response and adherence to medication; family history; presence of stresses; and others). In many cases the discontinuation of medication is not a simple process accomplished by simply saying, "No more pills starting tomorrow." Many psychotropic medications need to be discontinued gradually; some, over a period of a few days; and some, over a period of a few weeks (e.g., high dosages of alprazolam). Because polypharmacy has become quite common, discontinuation of medications could become quite a complicated task. Take an example of a patient treated with an antidepressant, a mood stabilizer, and a hypnotic. Which one should be stopped first? Second? We suggest that one never discontinue more than one medication at the same time. The sequencing of the discontinuation of several medications should be individualized, and all the general suggestions about discontinuation could be applied to each particular medication.

As Gabbard (2004) suggests, it is also important to assess the patient's readiness for termination. Although Gabbard's suggestion primarily concerns readiness to terminate long-term psychodynamic therapy, it may be useful to apply it in some cases of pharmacotherapy. The duration of pharmacotherapy for most disorders and conditions is a matter of consensus rather than a clearly determined period. The patient's readiness to terminate may be helpful in termination of pharmacotherapy also. It might be also very important to get input from family members or significant others on how the patient is doing.

The initial planning of pharmacotherapy termination should also include the discussion of what is going to happen with psychotherapy. The patient should clearly understand that terminating pharmacotherapy *does not* mean terminating psychotherapy (the resident should not forget that we are discussing the termination of pharmacotherapy while psychotherapy continues). Finally, the initial discussion may include the issues of recurrence of symptoms and follow-up after pharmacotherapy termination. However, these issues may come up more frequently during the process of termination itself.

Beitman et al. (2003) and others suggest announcing termination early, at least 3–6 months ahead. Mischoulon and colleagues (2000) also suggest the general timeline of 3–6 months for announcing the termination. They also provide several suggestions for ameliorating the change of psychopharmacologist, which may be adapted for termination of pharmacotherapy. These modified suggestions include informing the patient that symptoms may worsen transiently after the termination, reminding the patient of termination during each visit in the termination phase and allowing the patient to verbalize his or her feelings, and even using a standardized protocol for transfer and termination (Mischoulon et al. 2000). In cases of a transfer to a new psychiatrist, Mischoulon and colleagues (2000) also suggest that an early meeting with the new psychiatrist before termination with the previous one could be helpful.

We believe that the discussion of medication termination should also include further clinical issues such as the following:

1. The possibility of withdrawal symptoms (not only with benzodiazepines, but also with some selective serotonin reuptake inhibitors and other psychotropic medications) after stopping the medication. The discussion should include the timeline of these symptoms (e.g., withdrawal symptoms after the discontinuation of some benzodiazepines with long half-lives may be delayed for 1–2 weeks, whereas withdrawal symptoms associated with alprazolam may occur almost immediately) and a plan for their management.
2. The chance of increased suicidality during the discontinuation phase of some medications (see the recent U.S. Food and Drug Administration warning about the discontinuation of antidepressants) or after the discontinuation of lithium (e.g., Tondo et al. 1997).
3. Aftercare monitoring of withdrawal symptoms, recurrence symptoms, suicidality, and other clinical issues (which, in the case of continuing psychotherapy should not be difficult). In case any unusual symptoms occur, patients should be encouraged to contact the resident as soon as possible and at any time. Some residents may prefer being contacted via e-mail (for guidelines, see Silk and Yager 2003).
4. The possibility that patients may be offered an occasional medication review session after the termination (to check for possible relapse or recurrence). Or, if geography and time allow, the psychiatrist may step into a future therapy session if the need arises.
5. Avoidance of triggers of various symptoms. This means maintaining a healthy lifestyle, including avoiding or limiting the use of alcohol, caffeine, and tobacco; exercising; and getting regular and sufficient sleep.

Residents should always discuss the termination plan with their clinical and psychotherapy supervisors.

Competency: The psychiatry resident should be able to list specific issues to be considered when pharmacotherapy is terminated before psychotherapy.

All of these issues should be also discussed briefly with the nonmedical therapist. Both the patient and the nonmedical therapist should clearly understand that all medication-related issues during termination should be addressed with the resident. The therapist may face the patient's complaints and feelings of negative transference toward the resident (e.g., "She abandoned me") or dependence on the resident and medication (e.g., "I miss her very much"; "I cannot be without my pill").

It is important to emphasize boundary issues after treatment termination (Malmquist and Notman 2001). It should also be made clear to all parties that no medication will be prescribed beyond termination, if possible (Simon 2004). Residents themselves should also understand that termination really means termination. It is not appropriate to discuss any evolving or ongoing therapy issues after the resident has terminated pharmacotherapy. It is also not appropriate to give advice or discuss the pharmacotherapy after the patient has been transferred to another resident or primary care physician. Patients might call the resident and complain about the new clinician or solicit opinions about medication changes. These discussions should always be referred to the new clinician, and it may also be appropriate to let the nonmedical therapist or the new physician know about these contacts.

Terminating Psychotherapy First

Termination of psychotherapy in split arrangements while pharmacotherapy continues may occur fairly frequently. For instance, the patient underwent a course of brief psychotherapy for job-related stress during the ongoing treatment of recurrent major depression. Or there is simply nothing happening in therapy, and both patient and therapist feel that there are no more gains to be made and agree to terminate; however, the need for pharmacotherapy for a major mental disorder continues. Psychotherapy may be terminated after mutual agreement, but termination might be also unwanted, forced by various circumstances (lack of insurance coverage beyond a predetermined number of sessions, relocation of the therapist, etc.). Although the resident should be helpful in planning the termination of psychotherapy in split treatment, he or she may not be directly involved in its execution.

However, residents may frequently need to deal with the aftermath of psychotherapy termination. For instance, patients might express their negative feelings and doubts about the termination or negative transference toward their therapists. Some patients might attempt to continue therapy with the resident after the termination with their therapist. At times patients may develop negative transference toward their psychiatrist or become angry and openly hostile. They may question the reasons for continuing pharmacotherapy while psychotherapy is discontinued, especially when they have a strong bond with the therapist. Patients' negative feelings about termination of their therapy may also lead to nonadherence with pharmacotherapy. Also, psychotherapy may play a significant role in fostering adherence with pharmacotherapy (e.g., Pampallona et al. 2004). Once psychotherapy is over, patients may start to skip medication or stop taking it, either because the reinforcement provided by the therapist is missing or because of their anger and negative transference about the termination.

The psychotherapy termination is usually out of the resident's control. It is very important that the resident either be involved in termination planning or at least be informed about the planned termination. Psychotherapy termination in split-treatment arrangements should be carefully planned and individualized. The duration of therapy is frequently predetermined by the planned number of sessions, either agreed on at the beginning of therapy or forced by the third-party payer. Termination of psychotherapy should not only be discussed in psychotherapy but should also be briefly addressed during pharmacotherapy sessions. The resident might ask, "I heard from your therapist that you are going to terminate therapy soon. How do you feel about it?" Pharmacotherapy sessions may be used for some therapeutic support after the termination of psychotherapy or even for prevention of decompensation after the termination.

Just as in integrated treatment, the process of termination of psychotherapy may trigger various countertransference issues. A resident may overestimate pharmacotherapy or dislike the therapist. The resident's countertransference could hinder the proper planning and execution of psychotherapy termination. A resident may either fail to endorse the appropriate termination (Gabbard 2004) or overzealously endorse and force the termination of psychotherapy with the nonmedical therapist because it reinforces the resident's own rescue fantasies. Residents should avoid making inappropriate remarks such as, "Don't worry, you didn't need therapy anyway" or "It will be easy, you'll do fine on medication." In fact, residents should be aware that their countertransference may even trigger the termination of psychotherapy with the nonmedical therapist.

Residents might hold on to patients for their own needs (Gabbard 2004) and unconsciously sabotage the patient's treatment with anybody else. Residents should always discuss the termination of psychotherapy in supervision, even when they are not directly involved in its planning and execution. Any negative feelings toward the therapist or conflict with the therapist should be addressed in supervision as soon as possible. In training programs it is preferable that each party—resident and nonmedical therapist—address the conflict issues with their particular supervisor and the supervisor then attempt to resolve the issues with all parties involved. It is inappropriate and usually counterproductive to attempt to obtain leverage by involving only the resident supervisor. The nonmedical therapist may rightfully feel manipulated and ambushed and may refuse to collaborate on any solution. The patient is the one who ultimately suffers in such conflicts.

Termination of psychotherapy may also lead to boundary permeability. Gabbard (2004) addressed the increased permeability of boundaries between patient and therapist in a psychotherapy termination process. However, it is also possible that boundary permeability will expand into the pharmacotherapy process. Patients may ask the resident questions about the therapist or ask the resident to contact the therapist. The patient may try to leave a gift for the therapist with the psychiatrist. Patients may even ask the resident to intervene in the termination and stop it. Residents should be aware of the possibility that these boundary issues may arise. Some patients might also reveal to the resident that boundary violations with the therapist have occurred after therapy was terminated. These issues should be addressed on an individual basis in a proper framework and should be properly supervised. Residents should be aware that serious boundary violations (e.g., emotional or sexual involvement with the patient) are reportable to various authorities (e.g., ethics committees of professional organizations, legal authorities, the therapist's supervisor, or leadership of the treatment facility) and that residents may be required to report such boundary violations.

We recommend that the termination of psychotherapy in split treatment be well planned in advance and that it involve all three parties: the patient, the therapist, and the resident. Some guidelines for planning the termination of psychotherapy are listed below.

1. Termination of psychotherapy is planned and announced well in advance and the resident is informed about it from the inception of termination planning.
2. The patient's feelings, worries, and transference about and reaction to psychotherapy termination are regularly explored, discussed, and addressed in psychotherapy and also at times in pharmacotherapy. The patient should also be actively invited to verbalize his or her feelings about termination of psychotherapy during pharmacotherapy.
3. Possible decompensation, acting out, recurrence of symptoms, and occurrence of suicidality should be carefully monitored by the resident during the time of psychotherapy termination.

4. Adjustment or addition of medication may occasionally be offered to manage various symptoms or decompensation during psychotherapy termination. However, it should be made clear that these are temporary measures.

5. Increased attention to adherence to the originally prescribed medication regimen (i.e., continuing pharmacotherapy) is recommended.

6. Patients should be instructed to avoid stressors whenever possible during the termination of psychotherapy.

7. The resident should be aware of the possibility of increased boundary permeability during psychotherapy termination and that this increased permeability may extend to pharmacotherapy as well.

8. Frequent communication between the resident and the nonmedical therapist during the termination of psychotherapy is essential.

9. Residents should always seek proper supervision to address issues in termination of psychotherapy that may emerge during continuing pharmacotherapy.

> **Competency:** The psychiatry resident should be able to list specific issues to be considered when psychotherapy is terminated before pharmacotherapy.

Terminating Pharmacotherapy and Psychotherapy at the Same Time

Simultaneous termination of pharmacotherapy and psychotherapy in split treatment is probably infrequent. It may happen due to various circumstances and forces, which are usually outside of the treatment process. For instance, the patient could relocate, the third-party payer might force termination or transfer to another clinician or facility, the present facility may no longer accept the patient's insurance, or the treatment facility may close. At times termination of both pharmacotherapy and psychotherapy is forced when the patient does not show up for treatment. In such cases the patient is not terminating but is abandoning treatment. The treaters may be left with feelings and questions ("What went wrong?"), which may be addressed in discussions between the resident and the therapist and in supervision.

Simultaneous termination of pharmacotherapy and psychotherapy in split arrangement may stir up similar feelings as termination of both treatment modalities. Patients may feel angry, furious, abandoned, devastated, helpless, or hopeless.

Simultaneous termination of both pharmacotherapy and psychotherapy would require combining the recommendations about termination of both pharmacotherapy and psychotherapy (if the outside forces and time frame permit). However, we recommend avoiding simultaneous termination if possible because of the possible complications and difficulties associated with this process. Instead, we recommend sequencing the termination as discussed in this chapter, with the sequence being individualized and with the determination about the sequencing involving all three parties: the patient, the resident, and the therapist.

Simultaneous termination due to patient relocation, nonacceptance of insurance, or closure of the treatment facility requires proper referral whenever possible. The patient may be referred to a nearby clinic that will accept his or her insurance. The resident should provide a proper referral, including necessary telephone calls or correspondence. In the case of patient relocation, a proper referral is not always possible. The patient should be instructed either to contact his or her insurance representative in the new location, look up various facilities in the yellow pages, or contact the local university or a local psychiatric organization. The state psychiatric association and other organizations could be quite helpful in arranging referrals. The resident may offer direct help in making referral arrangements if he or she knows of a contact person or a colleague in the patient's new location. It is very important for the resident to try to facilitate such a transfer of care and to follow through on ensuring that the patient receives ongoing care. This is especially true for patients with psychiatric disorders of particular kinds and severities, such as psychosis, major depression, bipolar disorder, certain types of personality disorders, and substance use disorders and dependencies.

After the patient's proper written authorization for release of information has been received, the patient's record should be provided to other treaters (Simon 2004).

Simultaneous termination in split-treatment arrangements also requires addressing the posttermination boundary issues between the psychiatrist and the patient and between the therapist and the patient (Malmquist and Notman 2001). The probability and propensity for boundary violations are increased during the period of termination. Boundary violations may range from accepting expensive gifts to emotional or sexual involvement. The discussion of proper posttreatment boundaries should be always included in termination planning.

Conclusion

Termination does not necessarily mean the permanent ending of care. The patient may be explicitly invited by the resident, the therapist, or both to contact them in the future in case of setback or relapse.

Termination of treatment in patients with borderline personality disorder and other Cluster B personality disorders poses an especially difficult problem. Transfer from one resident to another in resident-staffed clinics has to be viewed and dealt with as a termination process in these cases.

Termination of either treatment modality may be introduced for clinical reasons (e.g., medication is no longer indicated, care is being transferred to another resident) or when the treaters (either one or both) feel that the collaboration is not working and they do not wish to continue working on the particular case together. This kind of termination should be done with a properly timed notice (so that a replacement for one or both treaters can be found) and after proper discussion (Gabbard 2001, p. 89) and careful supervision between the resident and the supervisor.

Patients may demonize the terminating clinician or try to manipulate the remaining clinician to assume the entire treatment (i.e., both modalities). Threats of suicide, self-mutilation, and other acting out may occur during the termination of one or both modalities and may pose a difficult and worrisome clinical problem for the remaining clinician. In addition, various accusations about the terminating treater may be divulged to the remaining treater. We have seen patients make statements such as, "After she told me too many things about herself, she wants to get rid of me"; or "We had such a close and intimate relationship and now he wants to get rid of me." These accusations have to be properly, yet very carefully, addressed in subsequent sessions.

As with the entire treatment, very strict limits must be set for termination of any treatment modality with patients with borderline personality disorder. It should be made clear that termination means termination and no further contacts are possible after the termination process has ended or after the patient has been transferred. One should remember that patients are very resourceful—in one example from our practice, a patient, after being transferred to a new resident, found the terminating resident (who had moved to another state for a fellowship) and started to call this former resident and make various demands.

Competency: The psychiatry resident should be able to list specific issues to be considered when pharmacotherapy and psychotherapy are terminated simultaneously.

References

Beitman BD, Blinder BJ, Thase ME, et al: Integrating Psychotherapy and Pharmacotherapy: Dissolving the Mind-Brain Barrier. New York, WW Norton, 2003

Bender S, Messner E: Becoming a Therapist: What Do I Say, and Why? New York, Guilford, 2003

Gabbard GO: Combining medication with psychotherapy in the treatment of personality disorders, in Psychotherapy for Personality Disorders. Edited by Gunderson JG, Gabbard GO (Review of Psychiatry Series; Oldham JM and Riba MB, series eds.). Washington, DC, American Psychiatric Publishing, 2001, pp 61–94

Gabbard GO: Long-Term Psychodynamic Psychotherapy: A Basic Text (Core Competencies in Psychotherapy Series). Arlington, VA, American Psychiatric Publishing, 2004

Makover RB: Treatment Planning for Psychotherapists: A Practical Guide to Better Outcomes, 2nd Edition. Arlington, VA, American Psychiatric Publishing, 2004

Malmquist CP, Notman MT: Psychiatrist-patient boundary issues following treatment termination. Am J Psychiatry 158:1010–1018, 2001

Mischoulon D, Rosenbaum JF, Messner E: Transfer to a new psychopharmacologist: its effect on patients. Acad Psychiatry 24:156–163, 2000

Pampallona S, Bollini P, Tibaldi G, et al: Combined pharmacotherapy and psychological treatment for depression: a systematic review. Arch Gen Psychiatry 61:714–719, 2004

Silk KR, Yager J: Suggested guidelines for e-mail communication in psychiatric practice. J Clin Psychiatry 64:799–806, 2003

Simon RI: Unilateral treatment termination: "You're fired." Psychiatric Times, July 2004, pp 25–26

Tondo L, Jamison KR, Baldessarini RJ: Effect of lithium maintenance on suicidal behavior in major mood disorders. Ann N Y Acad Sci 836:339–351, 1997

Part III

Evaluation, Monitoring, and Supervision

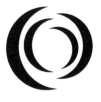

10

Evaluation, Monitoring, and Supervision of Integrated and Split Treatment

In the preceding nine chapters, we discuss how to acquire the necessary skills to become competent in planning and delivering integrated and split treatment. But how does one ensure that this educational process is heading in the right direction and that the residents accrue and ultimately possess the required skills and knowledge to competently practice integrated and split treatment? Residents' progress in acquiring these skills and knowledge sets has to be adequately and appropriately supervised, monitored, assessed, and evaluated. The competency has to be properly documented, not only because the Residency Review Committee (RRC) and the program reviewers will be looking for the ways competency in each area is documented. Rather, properly constructed documentation of this process will also allow training programs to properly structure the educational process and address deficiencies and other issues requiring change, improvement, and correction.

However, as Scheiber and Kramer (2003, p. 4) note, "Competence is not an all-or-nothing proposition. Competence is measured along a sliding scale through demonstrated knowledge and performed tasks. Competence is assessed by degrees. The measuring of medical competence has been a difficult activity. Just how much and exactly what must a physician know and be able to do to be judged 'competent'?"

What It Means to Be Competent

The first important question is what it means to be competent. In general, being competent means being well qualified, capable, and "having requisite or adequate abilities or qualities" (Merriam-Webster's Collegiate Dictionary 2003, p. 253). It also means being qualified or fit to perform a certain activity. Although being competent requires a certain level of expertise, it is not the same as being an expert. Most educators emphasize that being competent means achieving a skill level approximately midway between that of a novice or dilettante and that of an expert. The concept of defining, teaching, and evaluating or measuring competence (or competencies) is relatively new to medicine in general and to psychiatry in particular. There is little consensus in the field on exactly what it means to be competent in certain areas, and the operational definitions of what it means to be competent are slowly evolving. Being competent in integrated or split treatment means being qualified, knowledgeable, and skillful in integrating and combining two important treatment approaches (pharmacotherapy and various psychotherapies). It also means being knowledgeable of and skillful in providing these two treatments separately. In addition, being competent in split treatment means being skillful and capable in collaborating with other professionals (nonmedical therapists).

Combined Pharmacotherapy and Psychotherapy Competency Standards and Domains

Most of the authors and working groups that address the evaluation of competencies, including the RRC for psychiatry, suggest focusing on three domains of competency in various psychotherapies: knowledge, skills, and attitudes.

We chose to present the reader with two ways of summarizing the issues of competency in combined pharmacotherapy and psychotherapy. First, we provide the list of proposed competency standards or areas related to either integrated or split treatment as they are listed in the text of this book. Second, we summarize the competency issues according to the three domains: knowledge, skills, and attitudes. This briefer summary could be used for creating an assessment and evaluation form.

Proposed Competency Standards
Related to the Discussion in This Book

Competency Standards Related to Integrated Treatment

1. Psychiatry residents shall demonstrate an appreciation for the triage system that is in place at their institution for both inpatient and outpatient psychotherapy and psychopharmacological treatments. (Chapter 1, "Introduction to Integrated and Split Treatment")
2. The psychiatry resident should be able to demonstrate the ability to take a history regarding factors that would have an impact on the decision to provide the patient with split versus integrated treatment. (Chapter 1, "Introduction to Integrated and Split Treatment")
3. The psychiatry resident should be able to demonstrate the ability to ask questions regarding why the patient is being seen for a psychiatric evaluation (potentially medication and psychotherapy). (Chapter 2, "Selection of Medication and Psychotherapy in Integrated Treatment")
4. At the initial outpatient session, the psychiatry resident must demonstrate the ability to establish a doctor–patient relationship and to provide a trusting, warm environment to explore the patient's needs and problems. (Chapter 2, "Selection of Medication and Psychotherapy in Integrated Treatment")
5. During the evaluation phase, the psychiatry resident must be able to demonstrate the ability to develop a biopsychosocial formulation of the patient's problems; develop a problem list; and, together with the patient, develop treatment aims and prioritize the problems. (Chapter 2, "Selection of Medication and Psychotherapy in Integrated Treatment")
6. The psychiatry resident should, based on his or her evaluation of the patient, be able to select the appropriate combination of pharmacotherapy and psychotherapy. (Chapter 3, "Evaluation and Opening in Integrated Treatment")
7. The psychiatry resident should be able to discuss with and explain to the patient the selection of treatment modalities and their rationales. (Chapter 3, "Evaluation and Opening in Integrated Treatment")
8. The psychiatry resident must be able to demonstrate the ability to form a working therapeutic alliance at the beginning of treatment. (Chapter 4, "Sequencing in Integrated Treatment")
9. The psychiatry resident must be able to demonstrate the ability to appreciate the issues that involve sequencing of medication (other

medical treatments) and psychotherapy. (Chapter 4, "Sequencing in Integrated Treatment")

10. The psychiatry resident must be able to demonstrate knowledge of the factors that are important for the individual patient to maintain and adhere to a treatment regimen. (Chapter 4, "Sequencing in Integrated Treatment")

11. The psychiatry resident should be able to demonstrate the factors that are helpful in terminating care with patients. (Chapter 5, "Termination in Integrated Treatment")

12. The psychiatry resident should be able to demonstrate the skills and knowledge to terminate with patients regarding pharmacotherapy when both pharmacotherapy and psychotherapy were provided by the resident. (Chapter 5, "Termination in Integrated Treatment")

13. The psychiatry resident should be able to demonstrate the skills and knowledge to terminate with patients regarding psychotherapy when both pharmacotherapy and psychotherapy were provided by the resident. (Chapter 5, "Termination in Integrated Treatment")

14. The psychiatry resident should be able to demonstrate the skills and knowledge to terminate with patients regarding both pharmacotherapy and psychotherapy when both pharmacotherapy and psychotherapy were provided by the resident. (Chapter 5, "Termination in Integrated Treatment").

Competency Standards Related to Split Treatment

1. The psychiatry resident must be able to determine under what conditions split treatment would be most appropriate for a patient and be able to convey these issues to the patient. (Chapter 6, "Selection of Medication, Psychotherapy, and Clinicians in Split Treatment")

2. The psychiatry resident should be able to demonstrate the ability to determine his or her role in a split-treatment arrangement and to obtain the appropriate information from the patient, medical records, the referring therapist, other medical clinicians, family members, and other sources. (Chapter 6, "Selection of Medication, Psychotherapy, and Clinicians in Split Treatment")

3. The psychiatry resident should develop the ability to potentially reformulate a case. (Chapter 6, "Selection of Medication, Psychotherapy, and Clinicians in Split Treatment")

4. The psychiatry resident needs to demonstrate how to best terminate psychotherapy when both psychotherapy and pharmacotherapy are provided. (Chapter 6, "Selection of Medication, Psychotherapy, and Clinicians in Split Treatment")

5. The psychiatry resident must be able to understand the various dynamic and biological reasons for the request for a psychopharmacological consultation and be able to obtain the appropriate information to make an informed decision about the diagnosis and treatment plan. (Chapter 7, "Evaluation and Opening in Split Treatment")

6. The psychiatry resident should be able to determine the multiple issues that need to be addressed in the initial evaluation of a patient being referred by an outside therapist or physician, or as a self-referral. (Chapter 7, "Evaluation and Opening in Split Treatment")

7. The psychiatry resident must be able to balance the number of patients in split treatment with the complex and time-consuming nature of evaluating and treating such patients. (Chapter 7, "Evaluation and Opening in Split Treatment")

8. The psychiatry resident must be able to articulate and understand his or her role in the split-treatment arrangement: responsibilities, structure, and liabilities. (Chapter 7, "Evaluation and Opening in Split Treatment")

9. The psychiatry resident should be able to understand and perform a complete psychiatric evaluation of patients who are in split-treatment arrangements. (Chapter 7, "Evaluation and Opening in Split Treatment")

10. The psychiatry resident should be able to gather enough information to safely prescribe medication. (Chapter 8, "Sequencing and Maintenance in Split Treatment")

11. The psychiatry resident should be able to determine the factors that might make it judicious to provide medication at the first visit. (Chapter 8, "Sequencing and Maintenance in Split Treatment")

12. The psychiatry resident should be able to demonstrate that appropriate members of the patient's clinical team will know what medical care and medications are being recommended or provided by the resident. (Chapter 8, "Sequencing and Maintenance in Split Treatment")

13. The psychiatry resident must be able to determine when not to prescribe medication in a split-treatment arrangement. (Chapter 8, "Sequencing and Maintenance in Split Treatment")

14. The psychiatry resident should be able to demonstrate knowledge that the issues of maintenance of split treatment include termination issues. (Chapter 8, "Sequencing and Maintenance in Split Treatment")

15. The psychiatry resident should be thinking about and anticipating aspects of termination throughout all phases of split treatment. (Chapter 9, "Termination in Split Treatment")

16. The psychiatry resident should be able to list specific issues to be considered when pharmacotherapy is terminated before psychotherapy. (Chapter 9, "Termination in Split Treatment")
17. The psychiatry resident should be able to list specific issues to be considered when psychotherapy is terminated before pharmacotherapy. (Chapter 9, "Termination in Split Treatment")
18. The psychiatry resident should be able to list specific issues to be considered when pharmacotherapy and psychotherapy are terminated simultaneously. (Chapter 9, "Termination in Split Treatment")

These standards should provide residents, supervisors, and training directors with guidelines for thinking about, learning, teaching, and supervising competency in combined pharmacotherapy and psychotherapy treatment. The reader can quickly refer to the text to which each standard relates.

Competency Domains for Combined Pharmacotherapy and Psychotherapy

(We have used as a template the competency domains—knowledge, skills, and attitudes—for psychotherapy combined with psychopharmacology developed by the American Association of Directors of Psychiatry Residency Training; Sargent et al. 2001.)

Knowledge

At the end of training, the psychiatry resident should demonstrate understanding and knowledge of the following:

1. Diagnoses and clinical conditions that warrant consideration of psychopharmacological treatment in addition to psychotherapy, and psychotherapy in addition to psychopharmacology.
2. Different methods and approaches of combining psychotherapy and psychopharmacology (i.e., integrated and split treatment).
3. Specific indications for a recommendation of psychotherapy and psychopharmacology and the rationale for the type of psychotherapy and medication recommended.
4. Potential synergies and antagonisms in combining pharmacotherapy and psychotherapy.
5. The fact that taking medication may have multiple psychological and sociocultural meanings to a patient.

6. The background, education, and training of other mental health professionals who may provide psychotherapy in a combined treatment regimen.
7. Medicolegal and psychotherapeutic issues in the context of one person prescribing and one person providing psychotherapy: confidentiality, informed consent, and collaboration.
8. Understanding that continued education in combined pharmacotherapy and psychotherapy is necessary for further skills development.

Skills

At the end of training, the psychiatry resident should have acquired and be able to demonstrate the following skills:

1. Integrate biological and psychological aspects of a patient's history and other clinically relevant information to assess the need for, recommend, and implement integrated or split treatment (sequentially or simultaneously) in a mutually beneficial manner so that neither pharmacotherapy nor psychotherapy is neglected.
2. Complete the assessment for medication within the context of a psychotherapeutic framework while making interpretations and empathic comments.
3. Form an active alliance with the patient that facilitates adherence with both pharmacotherapy and psychotherapy.
4. Understand how the meaning of a medication to a patient can significantly affect its efficacy and learn how to explore the psychological and sociocultural meanings of medication to a patient.
5. Appreciate the potential psychodynamic issues of prescribing medication (resistance, compliance, and transitional object).
6. Use the placebo effect to prescribe medication more successfully.
7. Provide psychoeducation about medication in a manner that complements the chosen psychotherapy, appreciating the limitations of each treatment modality.
8. Identify and address the psychological aspects of nonadherence with medication regimens.
9. Use transference and countertransference and other psychotherapy techniques while prescribing medication to diminish resistance to medication and facilitate its use when appropriate.
10. Monitor the patient's condition and modify the pharmacotherapy or psychotherapy approach when necessary.
11. Appreciate and assess the importance of the timing of pharmacotherapy and psychotherapy intervention.

12. Recognize the ways that prescribing medication can enhance or hinder psychotherapy and the ways that psychotherapy can enhance or hinder pharmacotherapy.
13. Recognize and identify affects in the patient and in himself or herself.
14. Assess suicidality on an ongoing basis as it relates to the prescribed medication (or medications).
15. Be able to manage the termination process in both integrated and split treatment.
16. Recognize the patient's splitting between the resident and psychotherapist and address it in an appropriate manner.
17. Discuss the case regularly and collaborate effectively with the nonmedical therapist.

Attitudes

The psychiatry resident should be able to demonstrate the following:

1. Empathy, respect, a nonjudgmental and collaborative approach, and the ability to tolerate ambiguity and display confidence in the efficacy of combined psychopharmacology and psychotherapy.
2. Sensitivity to the sociocultural, socioeconomic, and educational issues that arise within the therapeutic relationship.
3. The ability to establish an honest and receptive educational alliance with the supervisor and incorporate material discussed in supervision into psychotherapy.
4. The understanding that the individual components of integrated and split treatment constitute the whole treatment and are not divisible into independent parts.
5. The ability to recognize obstacles to change and to understand possible ways of addressing them.
6. An ethical commitment to put the patient's needs before one's own (Gabbard 2004).
7. Acceptance of possible audio recording, videotaping, or direct observation of treatment sessions.

Evaluation and Assessment Tool

No uniform evaluation tool is available. We recommend that an evaluation tool or form be based on the three domains (knowledge, skills, and attitudes) to reflect residents' progress in the development of competency. For instance, the form could reflect whether a specific knowledge, skill, or attitude is not apparent, emerging, apparent, or well developed. An evaluation form could be a composite that serves as a summary of several cases (see "Requirements and Optimal Experience" below) or could be applied for each specific case used for competency training and evaluation.

We also recommend establishing a log of supervisory times and patient contacts. We found it useful and preferable for both the log of supervisory and patient contacts and the evaluation form to be kept by the competency supervisor (see "Requirements and Optimal Experience" below).

The evaluation form should serve as guidance during supervision of competency cases (see "Requirements and Optimal Experience" below).

Each program should also decide on the frequency of competency evaluations for combined (integrated or split) pharmacotherapy and psychotherapy (e.g., every 3 months or at the termination of a particular case, depending on whether a composite or a case-specific form is used).

Other tools that could be used for evaluation of combined pharmacotherapy and psychotherapy include videotapes, audiotapes, direct observation, presentations at case conferences, and write-ups.

Requirements and Optimal Experience

The optimal number of supervised and properly evaluated combined (integrated or split) pharmacotherapy and psychotherapy competency cases is difficult to define and depends on several factors, such as the availability of suitable patients and program caseload requirements for other psychotherapy competencies. The resident should preferably complete a minimum of six supervised and properly evaluated combined pharmacotherapy and psychotherapy cases during residency training. A minimum of three cases of integrated treatment and three cases of split treatment should preferably be completed during adult psychiatry training.

The exposure to cases of combined pharmacotherapy and psychotherapy should start fairly early during training, in some cases during the second year of training. The early start of competency training is especially pertinent for residents who plan to enter child and adolescent subspecialty training, because they may have to finish all aspects of their adult psychiatry training by the end of the third year of training. Optimally, combined cases could be spread through the second, third, and fourth years.

There is no optimal or best setting for treating patients using the combination of pharmacotherapy and psychotherapy. Inpatients and outpatients should be utilized for training of this treatment modality. However, the outpatient year of residency training may provide the most suitable grounds because the combined treatment could be executed in its entirety.

There are no specific selection criteria for selecting patients for combined pharmacotherapy and psychotherapy treatment. Each patient should receive individual evaluation regarding whether he or she is suitable for a combination of pharmacotherapy and specific psychotherapy. Residents should consult with a clinical supervisor on this selection process. However, we caution against selecting patients with an acute exacerbation of psychosis or acute mania as training cases for competency in combined pharmacotherapy and psychotherapy.

Supervision: Who, When, and How

Proper supervision is a crucial part of clinical teaching. However, one may ask, what are proper supervision, proper monitoring, good and competent supervisors, and a proper means of evaluation? The RRC requirements call for at least 2 hours of individual supervision each week. However, the requirements of competency in five core areas in various psychotherapies may actually press for more supervisory time. We advocate the use of separate expert supervisors for each competency (see below in this section). This may require a lot of juggling on the part of the resident to fit five supervisions into 2 hours, if the program adheres to having just 2 hours of supervision. Many residency programs provide for more supervision, frequently outside regular hours. However, even the extra supervision together with the regular supervision may not provide enough time for all therapies and clinical issues every week. Residents and supervisors might decide not to meet for supervision for each specific psychotherapy (cognitive-behavioral therapy, psychodynamic therapy, etc.) every week. They may arrange supervision for some modalities one week and for another on an alternate week. There might not be a need for supervision in some psychotherapies all the time; for instance, a resident may fulfill the requirements for brief psychotherapy (e.g., two completed cases) and will therefore need no further supervision specifically focused on brief psychotherapy. However, the supervision should occur fairly regularly and frequently.

We recommend that programs delegate specific supervisors with some expertise in each particular psychotherapy competency if the staffing level is sufficient to do so. This does not mean that one supervisor could not or should not be a supervisor in more than one competency if she has some expertise in both (e.g., brief psychotherapy and psychodynamic psychotherapy). However, in cases where one supervisor oversees more than one competency, specific supervision time should be devoted to each competency; the supervision of different competencies should not be lumped together.

Individuals who are assigned to supervise or oversee competency in combined (integrated or split) pharmacotherapy and psychotherapy should be seasoned, clinically oriented psychiatrists who are well versed in pharmacotherapy, at least one psychotherapy modality, and the combination and also in supervising and collaborating with other mental health professionals (reminder: the RRC also requires "supervised active collaboration with psychologists, psychiatric nurses, social workers, and other professional and paraprofessional mental health personnel in the treatment of patients"). Supervisors should keep in mind that becoming competent does not mean becoming an expert.

Proper individual supervision should address all three domains—knowledge, skills, and attitude—of the combined pharmacotherapy and psychotherapy competency. As Gabbard (2004) points out, there are different means of evaluation of competency (case write-ups, oral presentations at case conferences, written examinations, oral examinations, videotapes or direct observations, audiotape recordings, and individual supervision). The supervisor may select one or any combination of these for evaluating the resident. As Gabbard (2004) emphasizes, they all have certain advantages and disadvantages. However, individual supervision over time still seems the most useful in broadly evaluating all three competency domains. The newest way of evaluating competencies, an Internet-based examination, is in its infancy, and at this time no Internet-based examination for the evaluation of combined pharmacotherapy and psychotherapy is available. However, we have no doubt that such an examination will be developed in the near future.

Other means of evaluation, such as reviewing patients' charts and 360-degree evaluation (evaluation completed by several people, e.g., supervisors, collaborating nonmedical therapist, patient, patient families, colleagues, and subordinates), may be included to evaluate residents' competency.

Using a form developed on the basis of competency standards and domains and reflecting the progress of acquiring competency may be helpful in supervision sessions. Progress in addressing deficiencies could be effectively monitored and documented by the use of such a form.

A special area of supervision and evaluation in split treatment is the evaluation and supervision of collaboration with nonmedical therapists. Supervisors should monitor and address the content of communications between the resident and the nonmedical therapist. These communications should be regular and should not address crises only. Clashes and territory fights among professionals should be avoided and should be properly addressed in supervision when they do occur. Residents should properly collaborate with nonmedical therapists and should be able to discuss difficult situations with their collaborators. However, they should avoid direct confrontations, arguments, and especially conflicts in which patients are used as pawns in territory battles. Residents should discuss each difficult interaction with a nonmedical therapist during their supervision and should seek the supervisor's advice. Supervisors should avoid addressing conflicts between residents and nonmedical therapists without consulting and having supervisors of the nonmedical therapists involved or present. The same applies to supervisors of nonmedical therapists and seasoned nonmedical therapists. In the rare case of a serious conflict, a meeting between the resident, his supervisor, the nonmedical therapist, and her supervisor should be arranged to address and resolve the conflict.

Conclusion

Evaluation of competency in combined (either integrated or split) pharmacotherapy and psychotherapy is a critical part of developing a proper level of competency. It is a complicated task that requires adequate time, supervisory expertise, and the development of specific evaluation tools. Supervisors may decide to use one or more evaluation tools such as an evaluation form, a log of contacts, direct observation, oral or written examination, and case presentations at conferences. Proper evaluation should address all aspects, standards, and domains of competency, namely knowledge, skills, and attitudes. Special attention should be paid to the development of skills regarding how to collaborate with nonmedical therapists and other mental health and medical professionals and paraprofessionals.

References

Gabbard GO: Long-Term Psychodynamic Psychotherapy: A Basic Text (Core Competencies in Psychotherapy Series). Arlington, VA, American Psychiatric Publishing, 2004

Merriam-Webster's Collegiate Dictionary, 11th Edition. Springfield, MA, Merriam-Webster, 2003

Sargent J, Mohl PC, Beitman BB, et al: Psychotherapy Combined With Psycho-pharmacology Competencies. Farmington, CT, American Association of Directors of Psychiatry Residency Training, 2001. Available at: http://www.aadprt.org/public/educators.html. Accessed December 1, 2004

Scheiber SC, Kramer TAM: What core competencies mean to psychiatrists and trainees, in Core Competencies for Psychiatric Practice: What Clinicians Need to Know: A Report of the American Board of Psychiatry and Neurology. Edited by Scheiber SC, Kramer TAM, Adamowski SE. Washington, DC, American Psychiatric Publishing, 2003, pp 3–5

Index

Accreditation Council for Graduate Medical Education, 6
Adaptive history, 41, 100
Adolescents, psychiatric care of, 4, 5, 7
Adult psychiatry, settings for, 4, 7, 9–10, 22–25
Al-Anon, 57
Alcoholics Anonymous (AA), 27, 57
Alcohol use, 38, 97
Anxiety, treatment outcomes of, 1

Beck Depression Scale, 119
Biopsychosocial formulation, 27–29
Bipolar disorder, treatment outcomes of, 1

Caffeine use, 38, 97
Children, psychiatric care of, 4, 5, 7, 9, 10
Closed systems of care, 5
Cognitive-behavioral therapy (CBT), 44, 49, 54, 65
Collaborative treatment, versus split treatment, 2, 8, 83–84

Communication
    between residents and therapists, 26, 105, 107–108, 118–119, 125, 149–150
    boundaries and rules of, 69, 118, 129, 131, 132, 133, 134
    maintaining contact with patients, 24–25, 59, 118
Community mental health, systems of, 5, 6, 9
Comorbid conditions, factors impacting pathway of care, 4, 5, 7, 21, 26–27, 97
Competency
    attitudes and understanding as, 146
    demonstration of knowledge and skills in, 144–145
    evaluating residents' progress in, 146–147
    in integrated treatment, 6–7, 139, 141–142
    in psychotherapy, 6–7, 139–150
    in split treatment, 6–7, 139, 142–144
    measurement of, 139–140

Competency *(continued)*
   optimal experiences and
      requirements for, 147–148
   proposed standards and domains
      of, 141–146
   supervision of residents in,
      147–150
Confidentiality, 33, 87
Countertransference, triggers of, 4,
   62, 86, 114, 125, 130

Depression and Bipolar Support
   Alliance (DBSA), 57
Diagnosis
   as symbolic explanation, 45, 105
   DSM diagnostic classification of,
      7, 28, 43, 44, 102
   formulating of, 79–80, 102
   gathering information for, 32–43,
      84–102
   reassessing a working diagnosis,
      52–55, 102–103
Documentation
   in medical records, 33–34, 89
   in referrals, 77–81
   written consents of patients, 22,
      26, 107, 113, 133
Drug dependence, as comorbid
   factor, 26–27, 97
DSM diagnostic classification, 7, 28,
   43, 44, 102
Dysthymia, treatment outcomes of, 1

Educational history, 40, 99
Evaluation
   concerns and issues with split
      treatment, 83–108
   discussing diagnosis with patient
      in, 45–46, 105–108
   during first contact, 17–21, 31–35,
      87–103
   in integrated treatment, 31–43
   note taking during, 33–34, 89
   outline of information gathering
      in, 35–43, 93–102

psychiatric review of systems in,
   36–38, 95–98
Evidence-based practice guidelines, 1

Family history, 38–39, 98
Family meetings, goals for, 23
Financial resources of patients, 24,
   56, 66, 80, 129, 130.
   See also Integrated treatment;
   Split treatment
Follow-up, patient compliance with,
   20, 24, 105–108
Forensic psychiatry, 4, 7

Geriatric psychiatric care, 4, 5, 7, 9

Homicidality, 25, 36

Inpatient psychiatric care
   admission criteria and length of
      stay in, 8
   division of labor in care of, 8
   prescribing medication in, 22–23
Insurance providers, systems of
   mental health care in, 2–7
Integrated treatment
   assessing comorbid conditions in,
      25–27
   competencies in, 6–7, 139,
      141–142
   concerns and issues in, 17
   defined, 2
   discussion and opening phase of,
      45–46
   encounters/interactions as, 10
   initial call and evaluation in,
      17–21
   maintenance phase of, 55–56
   prescribing medication in, 21–25
   selecting treatment modality,
      27–29, 43–45
   sequencing of care in, 49–70
   simultaneous termination in,
      69–70
   termination of, 61–70

Internet, as resource for information, 22

Life stressors, 44, 103–104

Major depression, treatment outcomes of, 1, 62
Managed care, systems of mental health care in, 2–7
Marital history, 40, 99
Mental status examination, areas of, 41–42, 100–101
Military history, 40, 99

Narcotics Anonymous (NA), 57
National Alliance for the Mentally Ill (NAMI), 57
Nicotine dependence, treatment outcomes of, 1

Occupational history, 40, 99
Outpatient psychiatric care
prescribing medication in, 22–23
residency training in, 9–10

Patients
adherence and compliance with treatment, 37, 56–60, 103, 106–107, 124, 130, 132
education and resources for, 57–58, 92, 93–94, 106–108, 116–117
expectations of first sessions, 17–21, 31–35, 84–93, 105–108
factors affecting care of, 4–7
financial resources of, 24, 56, 66, 80, 129, 130
planning for termination of care with, 61–70, 124–134
written consents of, 22, 26, 107, 113, 133
Personal history, 5, 39–41, 98–100
Personality disorders, as comorbid factors, 21

Pharmacotherapy
adherence and compliance with, 37, 56–60, 103, 106–107, 124, 130, 132
financial considerations for, 24, 129, 130
history of previous treatment with, 21–25, 36–38, 96–97
in integrated treatment sequencing, 50–53
inpatient/outpatient settings of, 22–25, 114–119
in split treatment, 83–108, 123–134
length and termination of, 63–65, 116–118, 125–129
monitoring of, 23–25, 118–119
potential impact on patients' daily activities, 25, 104
side effects associated with, 25, 37, 56, 96, 104
Physical abuse, 39, 98
Primary care physicians
communication between residents and, 26, 105, 107–108
role in mental health care, 4, 96
Psychiatric residency
evaluating of competency during, 139–150
inpatient and outpatient settings for, 4, 22–25, 114–119
specialization within, 4, 7, 9–10
stages and training patterns in, 7–13
supervision during, 7–12, 75–81, 115, 120–121, 125, 130–131, 132, 146–150
Psychiatric review of systems, 36
Psychiatric triage
complexity and issues in, 2–5
professionals involved in, 2–7
Psychosomatic medicine, 4, 7
Psychotherapy
adherence and compliance with, 56–60

Psychotherapy *(continued)*
  areas of competencies in, 6–7,
    139–150
  developing biopsychosocial
    formulation for, 27–29,
    102
  evidence-based guidelines for,
    1–2
  in integrated treatment, 27–29,
    53–55
  in split treatment, 104–105,
    110–119, 123–124, 125
  length and termination of, 65–69,
    129–133
  problem summary list for, 28–29,
    102

Relational history, 40, 99
Residency Review Committee
    (RRC), 6, 139, 148, 149

Schizophrenia, treatment outcomes
    of, 1
Sequencing
  in integrated treatment, 49–60
  in split treatment, 109–119,
    123–124
Sexual abuse, 39, 98
Sexual history, 40–41, 99–100
Social history, 39–41, 98–100
Splitting, behavior of, 117–118
Split treatment
  combining treatment modalities
    in, 116–118
  competencies in, 6–7, 139,
    142–144
  formulating diagnosis and
    treatment plan in, 102–105
  initial evaluation and opening in,
    83–108
  maintenance phase of, 119–120
  ownership of care in, 87, 88, 92,
    93, 103–108
  patient education during, 92,
    93–94, 106–108, 116–117

prescribing/not prescribing in,
    103–105, 110–119
  role of resident in, 90–93,
    113–114
  scenarios/situations of, 75–81,
    83–108
  sequencing care and treatment in,
    109–119, 123–134
  specific concerns and issues in,
    83–108
  success of termination in, 124–134
  supervision during, 75–81, 115,
    120–121, 125, 130–131, 132
  versus collaborative treatment, 2,
    8, 83–84
Substance abuse/dependence
  comorbid factor of, 4, 5, 7, 26–27
  taking history of, 37–38, 96–97
Suicidality, assessing and monitoring
    for, 25, 36, 37, 64–65, 95, 96,
    112, 128, 131, 134
Supportive treatment, 49

Tardive dyskinesia, 51
Termination
  by patients, 61–63, 124–125
  discussing goals with patients,
    61–70, 123–134
  in integrated treatment, 61–70
  in split treatment, 123–134
  patient perceptions of, 61–70,
    119–120, 124–129
  posttermination boundaries with,
    70, 129, 131, 132, 133, 134
  residency rotation as form of,
    61–62, 66, 69–70, 119–120
Therapeutic alliance, forming during
    initial evaluation, 31–43, 83–108
Tobacco use, 38, 97
Transference, triggers of, 62, 118,
    125, 126, 131
Triage. *See* Psychiatric triage

University clinics, systems of mental
    health care in, 2–7, 9